What Others Are Saying About *The Four Stages of Yoga*

"In the tradition of all great storytellers, Nischala Cryer weaves thought-provoking tales, beautifully illustrating the intricacies, blessings, and challenges experienced in the four stages of life. Deeply inspiring."

>—Jamey and Darlene Potter, New Renaissance Bookshop,
>Portland, Oregon

"In a most engaging way, Nischala Cryer explains the traditional stages of a yoga practitioner's life by weaving into that paradigm the story of her own spiritual journey. She shares this journey, and deftly draws in the reader, by sharing fascinating stories and observations of her private interactions with some of today's spiritual leaders. She excites us with her tale, while simultaneously reminding us that, in truth, the highest journey is always to be found in our own heart.

"Highly recommended for both students and teachers of yoga. You will be entertained and educated with a soft and lyrical touch. Inspiring!"

>—Judith Hanson Lasater, PhD, PT, C-IAYT, E-RYT, yoga teacher
>since 1971, founding member of *Yoga Journal*, author of nine
>books including *Restore and Rebalance: Yoga for Deep Relaxation*

"You buy this book to figure out what to do with your kids. You keep reading, because suddenly it is about yourself. Then you want to give it to your parents, or your grandparents, but you can't, because soon you will become them and will need it yourself to guide your progress into, and through, the inevitable stages of life. This is a classic subject, but usually people write about it intellectually. I don't think it has ever been done in this how-to-live way. Entirely practical, with life-changing implications."

>—Asha Nayaswami, yogi in the fourth stage of life, author of
>*Swami Kriyananda: As We Have Known Him*

"Understanding the ancient wisdom of *The Four Stages of Yoga* is an essential asset to those treading the path of yoga. Thank you, Nischala, for your heartfelt clarity, which, when enhanced through stories, encourages us to celebrate each stage. Through the telling we are inspired to adapt the yogic practices to each stage, embracing spiritual enlightenment."

—Nischala Joy Devi, teacher, author of *The Healing Path of Yoga* and *The Secret Power of Yoga*

"The four ashrams, or stages of life, of Indian tradition have been virtually ignored by even the most ardent devotees of yoga and Hindu philosophy in the West, on the assumption that they are from a vastly different culture and a distant era. By presenting them as stages of yoga, or of spiritual development, Nischala Cryer has made a valuable contribution. Spiritual practitioners of all paths will find her framework practical, useful, and illuminating."

—Philip Goldberg, author of *American Veda* and *The Life of Yogananda*

"Ancient knowledge from the higher civilizations, when applied to everyday life, is reflected throughout this educational and entertaining book. An inspiring new contribution to the field of yoga, ideal for all ages!"

—Walter Cruttenden, Founder of The Conference on Precession and Ancient Knowledge (CPAK), author of *The Lost Star of Myth and Time*

"I love this book! The author's many life experiences and interviews with other yoga practitioners make for fascinating reading, marrying the most high-minded spiritual principles with a grounded life as a mother, wife, teacher, yogi, and nature-lover. Read this book! You will be inspired by her loyalty to her teachers as well as her expansiveness to truth-seekers of all traditions.

—Susan Usha Dermond, education consultant, former school principal, author of *Calm and Compassionate Children*

"This very readable narrative provides a firsthand account of life within a uniquely American spiritual community, seen through the developmental stages: learning, family, deep inquiry, and wisdom."

—Christopher Key Chapple, Doshi Professor of Indic and Comparative Theology, Director/Master of Arts in Yoga Studies, Loyola Marymount University

"Everyone loves a good story and *The Four Stages of Yoga* delightfully flows from one fascinating story to another. Nischala Cryer's fresh and fluid writing style brings each story to life, while she artfully weaves a gentle spiritual message into the narratives—a message rich in beauty and power because of the personal experience behind it. As an educator, I especially appreciated her insights into the first two stages of life. But no matter what stage of life you're in, whether you're new to yoga or a longtime devotee, you'll find inspiration here."

—Carol Malnor, MS in Education, co-Publisher and editor of Dawn Publications. author of eight children's books and the card deck *Nature's Portals: Inspiration through the Peace and Beauty of Nature*

"One of the first books that explains in detail what it means to live the four stages of yoga. The author gives an insightful description of lifelong education that this way of living entails. The author herself has been involved with such an education. This book is inspirational, scientific, and useful. You can use it as a guidebook if you are interested in integrating science and spirituality. An inspiring guide for life."

—Dr. Amit Goswami, quantum theoretical physicist, author of *The Self-Aware Universe*

"I hope you enjoy reading this as much as I did!"

—Savitri Simpson, author of *The Meaning of Dreaming* and *Chakras for Starters*

"This book offers the collected wisdom of a lifetime, and important insights to help anyone consciously use the natural rhythms of a lifetime for their own and others' spiritual benefit. You will find insights, practical suggestions, wise counsel, large-hearted humor, and accessible inspiration no matter where you are on your spiritual journey. Read it slowly and savor."

—Joseph Selbie, author of *The Physics of God*

"Through imaginative stories, true-life interviews, personal experiences, and ancient yogic wisdom, Nischala Cryer offers a vision of the purpose behind each stage of life. This book is a guide to living with fulfillment and enlightenment."

—Nayaswami Devi Novak, co-Spiritual Director of Ananda Sangha Worldwide, co-author of *Touch of Joy*

"This book is moving, entertaining, and full of wise insights for those engaged with yoga, nature, and the journey of life!"

—Joseph Bharat Cornell, Founder of Sharing Nature Worldwide, author of *Deep Nature Play* and *AUM: The Melody of Love*

The Four Stages

of

Yoga

The Four Stages

of

Yoga

How to Lead a Fulfilling Life

Nischala Cryer

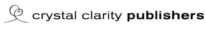

crystal clarity **publishers**

Nevada City, CA

Crystal Clarity Publishers, Nevada City, CA 95959

Printed in the United States of America

1 3 5 7 9 10 8 6 4 2

ISBN-13: 978-1-56589-310-8
ePub ISBN-13: 978-1-56589-569-0

Cover designed with love by Amala Cathleen Elliott
Interior designed by David Jensen
"The Land Between Two Rivers" illustration by Rose Ayala
"Astral Planes and Heavenly Abodes" illustration by David Jensen

---

Library of Congress Cataloging-in-Publication Data Available

℘ crystal clarity **publishers**

www.crystalclarity.com
clarity@crystalclarity.com
800.424.1055

To my guru, Paramhansa Yogananda, author of
Autobiography of a Yogi,
and to Swami Kriyananda, my teacher.

CONTENTS

Foreword, by Vanamali Devi 9

Introduction 13

"The Student" Birth to Age 24

1. The Student 19

2. Calling the Child 26

3. How Toddlers Teach Us 35

4. Yogic Schools for Youth 40

5. Girls' Rites 47

6. Boys' Rites 56

7. Ingrid's Message 63

8. When the Buddha Plays 66

9. When the Buddha Speaks 72

"The Householder" Age: 24–48

Illustration: *The Land Between Two Rivers* 84

10. The Householder 86

11. Gita's Way 89

12. How Couples Become 94

13. Family Yoga 98

14. Bhramachari Aditya 111

15. Nefretete 115

16. The Veil 121

17. Premabhava 126

"The Forest Dweller" Age: 48–72

18. The Forest Dweller 134

19. Wands of the Devas 138

20. Wild Things Are 146

21. Finding God in Nature 153

22. Brother Craig 160

23. Yogic Healing 172

"The Sannyasi" Age: 72–120

24. The Sannyasi 180

25. Mother Teresa 184

26. Yogis in Transition 191

27. Con Te Partiró 194

28. The Rishi 201

Illustration: *Heavenly Abodes & Astral Planes* 212

29. Death and the Astral Planes 213

30. Samadhi 223

Epilogue: Two Bears Crossing 226

Resources 230

About the Author 233

Foreword

By Mataji Vanamali Devi
Vanamali Ashram, Rishikesh, India

Nischala Cryer's *The Four Stages of Yoga, How to Lead a Fulfilling Life* is a unique book. It describes the four "ashrams" of Sanaatan* Dharma—Brahmacharya (the Student); Grihastashrama (the Householder); Vanaprastha (the Forest Dweller); and Sannyasa (the Sannyasi)—states or stages of yoga designed by the ancient rishis of India for a full and contented life.

Nischala has used a unique method of presenting these ashrams; she really comes at it from a novel angle. Instead of writing about these stages in an arid and uninteresting fashion, she has given us a vivid and graphic perspective of the topic by introducing some of the most unexpected and charming people who were living examples of these stages. She was fortunate to have met these people, studied with them, lived with them, and gleaned from their rich and varied experiences. Thus, she had a firsthand experience of what it means to be a modern yogi living in each particular ashram. She allows us a glimpse into the lives of these people, and places before us the essence of each particular phase of life through which all of us have to pass.

Whatever race, creed, or country we are born in, most of us pass through the first two stages—those of the Student (Brahmacharya) and the

---

* "The Eternal Religion." In *The Essence of the Bhagavad Gita*, Swami Kriyananda writes: "Sanaatan Dharma comprises those timeless truths which are rooted in eternity. They predate the forming of the world, and cannot be confined to any one earthly religion. Sanaatan Dharma embraces, indeed, all of manifested existence. Its manifestation in India is unlike other religions in that it was not a teaching by any one master, but expresses the essence of age-old, revealed wisdom." —publ.

Householder (Grihasthashrama). The next two stages of the Forest Dweller (Vanaprastha, or life of retirement from an active world), and the Sannyasi (complete detachment from the world), are rarely heard of in the West—or even in India, the birthplace of this concept. Very few people take advantage of or go through these latter stages today. Happily, this book illustrates the potential for experiencing these advanced states of yoga. The author has woven, around a cast of unique characters, a fascinating and beautiful tapestry of the stages of life which every yogi aspires to reach. The magic carpet of her words wafts us through delightful insights of the different stages of life, and eventually takes us to the threshold of the mystic door of death, through which everyone has to pass.

In the West in particular, there is a deep hunger to know more about the esoteric secrets of Sanaatan Dharma—the eternal order of right living, devoid of sectarian leanings or ideological divisions. This book will surely satisfy this desire and is a must for all lovers of yoga. It is written in a style appealing to Western readers and will surely open the door to further studies of these ancient teachings.

Hari Om Tat Sat

ACKNOWLEDGMENTS

To RAMA AND NAKULA, for your love, friendship, and support, I thank you every day. I am grateful for the editing expertise of Dayanand Salva and Nayaswami Prakash Van Cleve. Thank you to my walking partner, Laura Hermann; to Nayaswami Savitri Simpson; Anandi Gray; Chiara Lasagni; Mira Clark; and Rose Ayala. I would like to thank Seva Wiberg and Gloria Dunnagan for their cheerful friendship and for modeling the fourth stage of yoga. I am indebted to my teacher, Swami Kriyananda, for the expansive way he was able to bring into manifestation a yoga community that started as an experiment and now flourishes. I wish to thank Jyotish and Devi, for their sensitive community leadership and ongoing courage in modeling higher ways of living that we can all aspire to. For those who contributed to this book through interviews, many not recorded in these pages, I thank you. To all the students, householders, forest dwellers, and sannyasis, thank you for creating lives that inspire, uplift, and serve others.

Introduction

I was swimming in a lake on the Olympic Peninsula. It was summer, I was seven, and since the lake was about sixty feet deep, I was using an inner tube to stay afloat. I enjoyed being in the water and was having a pleasant time, so when I began to drift into deeper water there was no one around to observe me.

Noticing how far I was from land, I began to kick my feet within the inner tube hoping to get nearer to the shore. In my panic, the inner tube somehow came loose, and popped away from me, as inner tubes are known to do. I struggled to reach it. The combination of my fear and dog paddling could not catch it, so it drifted further away. The more I moved toward it, the quicker it seemed to escape.

I was now in very deep water. I could feel how much colder it was than the shallow water. Not having good swim strokes yet, I began to call out, but no one could hear me. My voice sounded tiny and the swimming dock seemed miles away. As I struggled to breathe and kick, my strength slowly ran out. Soon, my body went up and down, and I began to gasp both water and air.

I felt helpless. Each time I went down under the water, I became weaker and more scared. This continued for a while. My energy was leaving me. Finally, I began to sink farther down into the lake, and I could actually see the deep green water before my eyes. I remembered experiencing immense fear and panic.

As I sank deeper, I began to realize that I was dying. Further and further I sank. At some point, my mind accepted the fact of my death and I let go. *I am dying,* my mind repeated. Then, something unusual happened. The more I accepted my death, the more the fear began to leave me.

I was dying, and this was my journey. Since there was no longer anything to hang on to I began to embrace my death. Next, everything became exceedingly peaceful and calm, and there was a warm golden light that enveloped me. This field of light was so comforting and calming that I entered a state of bliss I cannot describe. I felt myself moving very quickly through light. The sounds I could hear were not external at all, but something I'd never experienced before.

There was no sense of time or space. I felt as though I'd been floating in this state for eons, thousands of hours, hundreds of years—or perhaps just seconds. The timelessness I experienced was so compelling that I instantly forgot about my earth life, my family, everything. I remember thinking *I love this place! I don't ever want to leave!*

How long this went on, I could not say. I learned later that my family, thinking I had already left the swimming area, had left too, and when they couldn't find me had returned. I awoke to find myself lying on the dock with people hovering above and calling to me.

Next, I recall feeling my body and the unpleasant sensation of water draining out of my mouth and nose.

It wasn't until I reached adulthood that I was able to process this experience, let alone talk about it. Young children, and even adults, can block things from their memories that are beyond their understanding or extremely unpleasant.

Over time, this experience began to sift through my consciousness.

It became a touchstone for me: *Do not fear the experience of death. It is really quite sacred.*

Years later, when I began to study yoga as my spiritual path, that experience finally made sense. I remember first hearing about the principles of reincarnation and yoga when I was twelve. It seemed like such a practical way to set up the universe. I just had to keep returning to the school of earthly life until I got it right, until I learned my lessons.

I came from a Christian household, so the rituals of church, youth groups, and sense of community were stabilizing factors in my early years. When my youngest brother was five, he was diagnosed with a rare bone disease and the doctors said he would never be able to walk. My mother was raised Christian Scientist and was influenced by Mary Baker Eddy, who drew her teachings from Hinduism. My mother had unshakeable faith in God.

I can still remember her gathering several of us together, telling us quite strongly, "Your little brother needs our prayers or he will never walk again!" I was about six. We all prayed, some of us wept, yet her energy was transformative. We couldn't afford hospital care, so my father and friends made a homemade traction device so that my brother could convalesce at home. All of us took care of him, pushing him in a wheelchair, the older brothers carrying him on their backs. After several years of prayers and love he was "miraculously" healed; he went on to play basketball and to lead a normal, healthy life.

At the age of twelve my relationship with Christianity was thwarted by my own internal questioning of the dogma that only the Bible and its translators could bring salvation. Didn't Christ say "In my Father's house are many mansions?" (John 14:2). It was not my intention to turn my back on Christ, I was seeking rather a deeper experience of God and Christ.

Around this time I found a book on yoga postures by a student of Ramana Maharshi. This was the late sixties, when American yoga was virtually nonexistent. I began practicing in the quiet of my tiny bedroom, with just enough space to do shoulder and head stands while occasionally crashing into the walls. The calmness I experienced following my yoga practices lifted me into meditative states.

We lived near the ocean in rural Cambria on the California coast. Most of my siblings were runners. We ran everywhere for play and recreation, and sometimes we ran barefoot. I could run from our house to the ocean in less than five minutes.

One day I discovered a hidden portal. It was about twenty minutes before sunset and I was running toward the ocean to find some driftwood. As I neared the water, something caught my eye and drew me closer. I'd already seen hundreds of sunsets, but this one was different. The roar of the ocean began to vibrate within my mind. I stumbled toward a huge log on the cliff above the rocky beach. My right arm reached down and felt it, touched it without taking my eyes off the scene ahead. I sat on the log.

Ahead of me the wild Pacific twisted and bobbed, a moving garland of sapphire and kelp. I gazed at the horizon, riveted. The orange globe descended from above like a slow-motion pantomime. Sky melted into the vast ocean. The roar of the sea belted through my mind and threw me out onto the horizon in an expanded state of consciousness.

Every day I vowed to visit at that exact hour, to dip into an altered state I could not verbalize.

In college my sculpture professor gave me a copy of *Journeys Out of the Body* by Robert Monroe. The book did much to explain what had been happening to me, beginning when I was quite young. My college dance instructor, a former *ballerino*, began his class with the Sun Salutation. I had some yoga in college, but back then, no one offered instruction in meditation.

I began working for UPI when I was nineteen, and before graduation inquired whether there was a job in foreign correspondence. A position was available in Beirut, Lebanon. I researched the number of journalists being killed there and quickly changed my mind. Well, the corporate world offered a safer salary. I could hide there!

Years later, when I read *Autobiography of a Yogi,* I was struck by the photo of Yogananda on the cover. His eyes were so deep, it was if he was looking right through me. I knew he had the answers I could not arrive at by myself. During one of my first meditations, using Yogananda's techniques, an image of Christ floated in my forehead, at the point between the eyebrows. This happened a few times, as if Jesus was reassuring me: *It's okay. We're all here together!*

In time I became involved with Ananda, a community of Yogananda followers practicing yoga and meditation. I was a founding member of their first urban ashram in the Bay Area, then moved to Ananda Village after I met Nakula, who'd been a follower of Yogananda since 1969.

When the founder of Ananda, Swami Kriyananda, was a young man, he had lived with Yogananda. Years before, Yogananda had formed a monastery; now he put Kriyananda in charge of the monks. Sometime after Yogananda's death, Kriyananda left the organization.

Kriyananda became my teacher and performed the marriage ceremony for Nakula and me in 1990. We had a son named Rama, and twelve years later, Nakula and I founded a small college, Ananda University.

In 1998, when Rama was a young boy, we took him to Assisi, Italy where my teacher was living. I had just published my first book, *Reflections on Living 30 Years in a Spiritual Community*. During a meeting in Assisi I interviewed Kriyananda for a book on the Four Ashrams of Life, the foundation for this book. As was his nature, my teacher gave me an astute and thorough interview. It has taken twenty years to absorb what he told me that day.

After Yogananda's passing, my teacher visited India many times. He became friends with many saints and sages. He spent time with Anandamoyi Ma and other great masters. He met and spoke with the Dalai Lama shortly after His Holiness had escaped from Tibet to India. He befriended the female mystic and author Vanamali Devi, who still lives in her small ashram in Rishikesh. The two often communicated, and shortly before my teacher died, Vanamali had the intuition to visit him in Pune, India. "It was the last time I saw him alive," she said.

Yogananda's mission to bring yoga to the West was heralded by the great spiritual master Mahavatar Babaji. As chronicled in Yogananda's classic *Autobiography of a Yogi*, the deathless Babaji said that the spirituality of India, when combined with the practicality of America, would lead to the creation of a more balanced society.

In 2016 *Yoga Journal* conducted a study with Yoga Alliance and reported that the number of yoga practitioners had increased to more than thirty-six million. They also noted that 34 percent of Americans, or eighty million people, said they were likely to try yoga for the first time within the next twelve months. That was several years ago, and the numbers are still rising.

Today, yoga practice and instruction are helping people live healthier, longer lives. The teachings of Vedic India, as revealed in this book, open the door for deeper experiences of the yoga Yogananda originally brought to the West in the early twentieth century. Yogananda's teachings on yoga are in harmony with scientific knowledge, and filled with profound meaning.

In the higher civilizations of the ancient past, the Indian rishis established "four ashrams," or ways to live during the four principle stages of life, that offered a remedy for societal ills. Modern-day communities and those of the future have the potential to fulfill many noble traditions passed down from higher civilizations. Although their outward manifestation may be uniquely adapted for each situation, if they help people to nurture and develop their inner lives from birth to death, they can be a great boon to society. Through this book I hope to re-awaken knowledge of these benefits and show how they can be applied by all.

CHAPTER 1

The Student—Birth–Age 24

Prelude

IN THE HIGHER CIVILIZATIONS, the rishis established a path that led to the heavens.

Along the path were four stations. Inside the stations were remedies that helped people lead more fulfilling lives. There was the Student Stage, encompassing birth to age 24; the Householder Stage, for those 24 to 48; and the Forest Dwellers, for those 48 to 72. From age 72 to 120 came the last stage, the Sannyasi.

To illustrate the four stages of yoga, a few of my stories are fiction, the essence of which are drawn from the Vedic culture of Hinduism. Some of these stories contain symbols with esoteric meaning for yoga adherents. I also share episodes from my own life in a yoga community where people strive to live spiritually conscious lives. There are interviews with those who have lived in these four stages. And, like the following fiction story, there are visionary depictions of what a yoga community in a higher civilization might be like.

A CRESCENT MOON IS FLOATING high in the sky. In the east, the sun is slowly awakening. A group of people gather at a mountaintop retreat to watch the sunrise. Below the canyon a river moves quickly. The congregation finds seats among the leaves and grasses.

Musicians gather, carrying stringed instruments, flutes, bells, and harmoniums. Lively notes rise as the players attune to each other, listening without speaking. Through their wisdom they will teach music and songs, the yoga of magnetism, and attunement to subtle energies. There is clapping, drumming, and the sound of tiny kirtals ringing together as the children's band enters and joins the musicians. They are followed by a barefoot procession of youths carrying an assortment of drums.

Before the crowd an earthen stage overlooks the river. Approaching the stage are elders, their locks grey and white, their eyes filled with wisdom. They are adorned with garlands of springtime and in their hands, they carry conch shells of all shapes and size. The orchestra begins to play, the elders move about the stage, their robes glowing with light. The music stops. The elders raise shells to the heavens, and each in their own time blows their sacred conch. Again and again the conch shells sound, the trumpeting varied and piercing. The elders are smiling and laughing, a light mood uplifting the entire gathering.

More elders surround the stage, bedecked in luminous garlands that reach beyond their knees, swinging gently as they move. Each garland is uniquely colored, handmade by the coveted costume designers who dress and bless them for the occasion. The gathering crowd includes children, youths, families, monastics, neighbors, parents carrying babies, and well-wishers from nearby communities. All have joined on this blessed day to welcome the students.

The elders fold their palms together in prayer, and, facing the sun, begin the Sanskrit recitation of the holy Gayatri Mantra. They continue for an auspicious number of times, aware that the children are restless, their energy unbounded and awakening.

A choir assembles next to the stage, singing as the elders lightly dance, prelude to an event everyone will join. The elders exit, eyes glowing with calmness, still swaying, some with palms folded close to their hearts. The elders watch. Their energy is a vital source of well-being to the students. They will teach the students meditation and yoga, mantras, rituals, dances, and songs. The children will learn how to make costumes and how to grow their own food through their work in the gardens. They will learn how to master a craft or start a business, use yogic healing techniques and learn how to live in harmony with all. In return these students will someday care for their elders with the same love and energy they have been given.

From the orchestra come the drums, primordial rhythms ascending from the earth itself, awakening and directing the energy of the songs. Their beat represents the progression of creation, from the beginning to the present moment. A barefoot man with long flowing hair, a beatific smile rising from his mouth, enters the crowd, his hands striking a small drum he holds in the air. His skin is bare and tinged a slight blue, the color of the morning sky. He is muscular, his physique like that of a Vedic god, his gaze forward yet inward. His inner left forearm features the tattoo of a large flame representing the destruction of the old and the beginning of the new.

His right hand holds a *damaru*, the hourglass drum symbolizing the dynamic blend of male and female principles. With his drum he creates the rhythm of life that keeps civilizations moving and dancing. With his left hand he points downward to the demons he has overpowered, symbolizing his ability to conquer the lower forces of delusion that prevent one from recognizing the Higher Self. His right palm faces outward in a gesture of blessing to all.

Around his neck are garlands that twist like shimmering snakes of red and gold, obsidian and earthen brown, signifying his perfect detachment. They intertwine with heaps of prayer malas noting his dedication to meditation. In the middle of his forehead, a third eye given him by Parvati, mother of his son Ganesha, lies closed, allowing his bodily form to remain on the earth plane unfettered. His dhoti is that of an ascetic, befitting "the King of the Yogis." The dance of Shiva begins.

Shiva's dance symbolizes the ecstasy of yoga and divine states of union. His movements guide the cycles of time. Bending his knees and lifting his left foot off the ground, he pauses, facing the children and their parents, the teens and the young adults. Their eyes light up, their breath pulls inward in disbelief. Were it not for Shiva's calm inner joy they would be terrified. He twirls and leaps around the earthen stage, each step stronger, bare feet hitting the ground, his long hair vibrating out.

After the invocation a troupe of young men join Shiva's dance, mimicking him, swirling and shifting with timed precision. They use muscular body movements and hand mudras, joining in a yogic dance that thrills and entertains. There is laughter, clapping, music. Now other male dancers enter, the youngest following his elders, imitating their movements. Like Shiva their skin is bare from the waist up, adorned with garlands of prayer malas. They are dressed in loose golden pants that flow and swirl enhancing their athletic, graceful, and meaningful gestures.

The music shifts to include the waiting stringed instruments, flutes, and harmoniums, while the drummers continue to define the dance, their hands setting the sensitive pace. A chorus of male voices filled with devotion and longing sends a clear message: *"Namo Shivaya, Namo Shivaya, Hari Hari Bol, Hari Hari Bole, Nama Shivaya."* Their pleas are answered by a group of women singers, calling to Shiva from their hearts.

Some say the earth is female, and energy is male. Others say the earth is male, the energy female. Like the hourglass shaped drum that Shiva carries, both energies are necessary.

More dancers enter the scene: women in graceful iridescent saris, their harmonious forms enhancing an atmosphere of deepening energy and movement. They are followed by barefoot female youths in colorful costumes. They dance the symbols of Shiva with intricate hand and body movements. Each movement of their eyes, brows, facial expressions, and necks signals a subtle but profound story acknowledging the path of yoga.

All the congregation dances, the toddlers giggling hand in hand, while parents carefully rock their babes. The dance draws to an end. A loud temple gong rings seven times, echoing throughout nature, penetrating the ether.

A divine wind blows gently, obscuring the view and causing everyone to sit and close their eyes. Gentle music floats in with the wind, then stops. All movement ceases as if nature itself has cast its last stone. The quiet inward breathing of Shiva, the King of the Yogis, holds the group in a meditative state.

Afterwards, the crowd rises and files towards an attractive circular temple honoring all of the world's religions. In the center of the temple, buried beneath the ground, resides a copper Sri Yantra, a yogic symbol from higher civilizations containing the sacred geometry of the universe. Inscribed in the middle of the Sri Yantra are symbols to strengthen the positive energy of the temple.

The crowd walks around the temple clockwise three times, their movements slow and meditative, their hearts receptive. The Sri Yantra beneath the temple acts as a conductor, absorbing earth's magnetic waves and radiating high vibrations outward to the surroundings. It continues to emanate energy in concentric circles, and when a temple bell sounds, the energy whorls expand further beyond the temple. The sensitive devotees circumambulating the temple are engulfed in this energy field, receiving more benefits the more times they circle. Some of the youth complete the circle 108 times; others prostrate themselves, the entire front of their bodies touching the ground in an act of total devotion to God, thus receiving not only the temple's vibrations but emanations from the earth itself. The energy from the temple continues to spread outwards in circles like waves in a pond, the vibrations building more and more each time it is circumambulated.

Inside the temple the elders migrate to the front of a beautiful altar in honor of spring. Before the altar is a large copper bowl filled with rose petals blessed during a sacred meditation ceremony. Mixed in with the rose petals are prayer malas that the students will receive to encourage their noble meditation efforts. The malas each contain 108 beads of a special kind, known to hold the sacred vibrations of meditation. The students who are ready to receive the blessings arrange themselves in single file, and, one by one, approach the altar, kneel with their hands together, and await the elders who step towards them.

Each elder has been preparing to bless the students. Separately, and in small groups, they have been meditating and singing to the Infinite for this special event—the Blessing from the Elders. All are dressed in their finest robes, and each is carrying a secret blessing they will share.

As the elders stand in front of each student, they join their palms in *namaste*. Through their years of yoga practice they have gathered much knowledge and love. Now they will reach out and bless each student at the heart chakra, or at the point between the eyebrows: the third eye of intuition. They continue until each student has been blessed, a ceremony held each year on an auspicious day to honor the students.

It is spring. The yellow daffodils are pushing through the damp ground. High in an oak tree, a pair of doves call to each other. The song of a cheerful robin fills the air with excitement. An urgency can be felt. The youthful energy is boundless, uncaptured.

Nearby, a small temple school stands waiting. Outside, a group of young friends are discussing the nature of consciousness, and of God. "How can you prove that Spirit exists?" one asks. Another replies, "How can you explain the unexplainable?' A third youth answers, "If you've never seen something unbelievable, how can I explain it to you if your mind is not able to accept it?" Then, another student joins in, "If I told you that time and space are illusions and that yogis have traveled to other dimensions would you believe me?" Silence. "Probably not," one replies.

And so it is. We can only understand that with which we've had a personal experience or are willing to acknowledge. We know that living things are born, grow, and then die because they are physical manifestations. We can read about spiritual experiences and wish to discover more about them, yet until we've experienced the unexplainable ourselves, to our minds they remain in the realm of myth. The reason people are intrigued by myths is, somewhere deep in their consciousness, their souls remember something they cannot articulate.

The great female saint Anandamoyi Ma, whom Yogananda referred to in his classic *Autobiography of a Yogi* as "the Joy-Permeated Mother," knew the benefits of the four "ashrams" or stages of yoga. She saw them as a way to bring into manifestation important values from the ancient sages of India that would add stability to society. "Only if young people are taught self-control, even-mindedness, unselfishness, and God-centeredness, would they be well-grounded in the art of living,'" she said. She advocated for brahmacharya, in which young men and women would live a celibate life and receive training from their spiritual mentors before embarking upon the householder path.

In the middle of the temple school a statue sits stoically in the lotus posture, eyes closed, his left hand turned upward on his inner thigh. His right hand is gently raised outward in blessing to all. To his right rests a long trident. On his forehead, between his eyes, a small crescent moon pulsates with light making his blue skin appear supernatural. His long hair weaves around and around his head in a snakelike gesture, and draped around his chest are prayer malas. His silence and stillness are a physical force helping all go deeper into the asana of meditation. Sitting next to him is his wife Parvati, the embodiment of the spiritual energy known as "shakti." On her lap rests their son.

Outside the temple, a golden striped tiger kitten lounges, licking its paws, its green eyes studying the scene with alacrity.

---

* Alexander Lipski and Anandamayi Ma, edited by Joseph A. Fitzgerald, *The Essential Sri Anandamayi Ma* (Bloomington, Indiana: World Wisdom, 2007), 72.

Chapter 2

A child is born on that day and at that hour when the celestial rays
are in mathematical harmony with his individual karma.
—Swami Sri Yukteswar, *Autobiography of a Yogi* (1946 edition)

Calling the Child

D URING THE MONTHS AND weeks leading up to our son's birth we thought of many things that most parents consider, like, what shall we call him? For several reasons, our baby doctor had recommended an ultrasound, so we knew we'd be having a boy.

The naming process resembled a game of badminton. We'd each write down names and vigorously defend our positions. We'd had several months to play, but there still wasn't a winning title. As our son was born three weeks early, we stopped focusing on the name we might give him. Thus, when the nurse came into our room to ask what his name would be, we both looked at each other blankly, knowing that this was not the time for badminton.

I was holding our son, now just twelve hours into this earthly incarnation, when a new name bounced into my mind. "Rama," I said. "What do you think of the name Rama?" To my surprise, my husband, Nakula, answered, "Yes, I like that name." It was the easiest naming session we'd had. When I reflected on that scene, it was as if this little one had given us his own name right from the start. It was an easy name to remember, not too complicated or difficult to pronounce, and we gave him two additional names, should he wish to use an English name in the future. Later, when he was old enough to comprehend, we told him about his name and how it had come to us. Rama was a name that stuck. He has not changed it, and seems content with it.

When Rama was around eight, I read to him from *Watership Down* by Richard Adams. The characters are mythical rabbits with charming names and personalities. The book is somewhat of an allegory of the struggle between oppression and freedom. There are subtle undertones of ecology and habitat protection that weave throughout the story.

Sadly, when our son was nine, two of his best friends left the yoga community we lived in and moved far away. My son pined for them and asked when he would see them again. I told him that when he and his friends were older, they would look back on their youth, and their secret code would be the Sanskrit names they all had carried at that time—much in the same way the mystical rabbits in *Watership Down* had secret names from their youth.

Names and the naming process hold a much deeper reality, as Swami Jnanananda (pronounced "Gyan-ananda") Giri once pointed out to me during a gathering at his tiny home in Dehra Dun, India. I had just received the Sanskrit name I'd waited nearly twenty years to adopt. The name had come to me during an eight-hour meditation, broadcasting itself after a period of deep prayer. After my meditation experience I had asked my own teacher about it, and Kriyananda confirmed that the name was an excellent choice. Very few people knew I'd been given a name.

In retrospect, I had many interesting experiences with Swami Jnanananda. And now, here we were, taking a group of college students to visit this saintly rishi in India. As we often did when we were with him, we listened. He rarely spoke, and when he did, chose his words carefully. After we had been chanting and meditating with him, he looked at me and said in a very loud voice. "Never forget the name you were born with, for it has meaning too." He continued to look at me rather sternly, peering right through me and reading my mind. He explained his own given name, and the meaning and symbols attached to it. My birth name had been Sara, which is like the Sanskrit name

Saraswati, the appellation for the goddess associated with education. There was already one Saraswati residing in our yoga community in California, so it never occurred to me to want that name. Jnanananda's point was to show me that nothing is a mistake, that often the subtlety of a birth name can determine a calling or dharma.

The Indian scriptures speak of the "yugas," or great cycles of time—eras through which human civilizations rise and fall. According to Yogananda's guru, the great saint of wisdom, Sri Yukteswar, in these yogic cycles of rising and descending consciousness, we are now in the very beginnings of ascending Dwapara Yuga: the Age of Energy. Now, therefore, the Vedic history of names has more significance, in that we are moving upward in our ability to understand consciousness and its impact in our daily lives.

Many early Vedic texts prescribe more than one name for an individual. According to the Rig Veda, a child of either sex should be given four names, including the Nakshatra name (according the constellation the child was born under), the name of the deity associated with that month, the family deity, and another, popular deity. In the East, the Hindu naming process is very precise.

Directly after a Hindu birth, a special prayer is offered and a mantra chanted offering peace or the generation of talent. This is sometimes the moment when the father welcomes and blesses his child with a small taste of ghee. Ghee is clarified butter and often used in sacred ceremonies, a touching tribute that reaffirms the father's commitment to supporting the child's growth on all levels, especially spiritually.

The naming process is held during the tenth and forty-first days of life. Names are chosen according to astrology, and names of gods and goddesses are chosen as an added blessing. Other points to consider include a name that's easy to pronounce and pleasant to hear, and perhaps one that offers positive attributes.

Many Westerners have been given names that originated from Christianity, Judaism, or other belief systems. In our case, and possibly this is true for many in the West, our child and the universe seemed to suggest a name ideally suited to his own life.

In the yoga community I've lived in for the past thirty-three years, we observe a number of rituals that can help parents bring a soul into their family. The most important ritual is that of daily meditating with your spouse. When two people meditate together, they create a magnetism that will eventually draw to them a soul of harmonious nature.

Through meditation a nonverbal communication takes place that allows young parents to attune and harmonize themselves on a deeper spiritual level. Some parents wait several years before having a child, and some conceive fairly early on. There is no right or wrong, but an established meditation practice helps greatly.

The child you're hoping to attract dwells on the astral or energy plane of existence. They will be magnetized to you based on the individual karmas and vibrations of your family. Together, a couple offers prayers for a harmonious child, especially during the months just before planning to conceive.

In the book *Conversations with Yogananda,* Swami Kriyananda relays instructions Yogananda had given to a family he was helping to draw a specific child into their lives:

"A couple expressed to me their desire for a spiritual child. I prayed for them, then showed them a photograph. This soul, I told them, would be suitable for them, and was also, I felt, ready to be reborn on earth.

"'Meditate on this soul,' I said. 'Concentrate especially on the eyes. Invite him to come dwell in your home. In addition, have no sexual contact for six months; abstinence will increase your magnetism.

"'When, at the end of that time, you come together physically, think of that person, and think also of God. If you follow my advice in all these respects, that soul will be born to you.'

"They followed what I'd told them, and, some time later, that was the very soul which was drawn into their home."*

Lest any couples find it difficult to follow these guidelines, remember that Yogananda, as a spiritual master, was in this instance offering specific advice to one particular couple. Over the years I've asked couples in our yoga

---

* Swami Kriyananda, *Conversations with Yogananda* (Nevada City, California: Crystal Clarity Publishers, 2004), 204–5.

community if they had been able to follow these guidelines. Most said that they had prayed in advance for a spiritual soul to join their family, one who would be harmonious within their family.

One mother told me that she and her husband had been trying for a few years to conceive and without success. She began to think that maybe they weren't supposed to have a child. While meditating on whether they should cease trying, she was astonished to hear a chorus of voices saying, "No, no. There's a soul coming. Don't give up." After this experience, she conceived within a few months.

Our goal as parents is to grow to understand, on a deeper level, the meaning of love, and to try to act as pure channels of love and higher consciousness in this world. The cradle of love that we create in our hearts will draw the right children to our families.

It is our own karma as parents and as a family that draws a soul to us. If your child is born handicapped, this is grievous and can be a challenge to all involved. But is it, on every level, a misfortune? Yogananda once said that a man who was born a spastic was actually very near to God-realization; he was just finishing off the last threads of his karma. The experience of raising a challenging child can be good karma. Through the process, one can build inner strength and character. As Yogananda once said, "A smooth life is not a victorious life."

Bringing a child into the world is one of the most important decisions two householder yogis can make. When a man and woman come together sexually, when the sperm and the ovum unite at the point of physical conception, a light is generated in the astral world. Souls that resonate with that light and are ready to be born will be drawn to it. My teacher once said that these souls may not necessarily be inside the womb yet. In the cases of twins or multiple births, more than one soul was attracted to that light.

Love is a powerful magnet, so certain souls with close attachments to others, past relations especially, might naturally choose to come back, if possible, and be near them again. Souls reincarnating with past family members and friends is not uncommon. The reincarnating soul may also have been part of a group of spiritual people it feels close to and wants to return to earth to join them.

According to the great yogis, the earth plane is the best place to work out karma because it's easier here. On the higher astral planes, our ability to create can be instantaneous. The weather there is perfect, the scenery ideal, the people all loving, and it really is quite heavenly. Our souls can remember this state, a reason we long to recreate harmony, peace, beauty, and love here on the earth plane.

In our yoga community we greet babies before their actual birth, to express our support. We hold gatherings with prayers, music, and a celebration in our temple. Often the mother or parents are both seated near the altar. We come forward and kneel in front of the parents. We pray for and send loving energy to the new soul and to both the parents.

Once, a young friend of ours whispered to me the news. She and her husband planned to adopt a baby and asked for prayers in this endeavor. After they received their beautiful child I asked her approximately when the date was that she and her partner had seriously considered adoption. She said it was during our annual Spiritual Renewal Week, considered a sacred time for the community. The child they were given was born exactly nine months from that time. Adopted births are just as predestined as any other birth.

Before delivery, couples select the type of birth they feel would be best for them and their child. Many choose home or water births. In our case, my husband wanted a home birth. My intuition said to have a hospital birth, something not many couples in our community were opting for. Later I understood why. Our son was born with congenital heart defects that could have been fatal if left unattended or if not diagnosed by a trained medical doctor.

Our nurse was checking Rama in the wee hours after his birth. Shortly thereafter I heard a tense and excited conversation between medical staff. They were checking his heart. The next day, instead of going home, we traveled to a larger hospital and our baby received tests that confirmed his condition.

If I hadn't listened to my intuition the sophisticated test needed to help Rama and schedule a surgery wouldn't have been available. I was grateful for the medical doctors and humbly understood that God certainly worked through physicians too. So much has been said against Western medicine, yet we are in a time of transition when we need to work together as more advanced healing methods are adopted.

For the first month after a new baby is born in our community, we support the family with home-cooked vegetarian dinners, prepared by community members. It's a gesture of love and an opportunity for us to meet the new child and offer our blessings.

The greatest gift we received, though, was extraordinary. During the eight hours our baby was having open-heart surgery, the woman who later became principal of the Living Wisdom School led a prayer vigil. With close to two hundred people in the community meditating and praying for Rama, the surgeons and both of us felt uplifted and calm. When the doctors spoke to us after the operation they expressed their amazement. Rarely had they seen a baby look so vibrant following a surgery for his condition.

Coincidentally, the principal's spiritual name was Hridayavasi, which means "the Lord dwelling in the heart." She once told me that, when she was given that name, she felt an instant attunement with it. Often these Sanskrit names offer beautiful qualities or present an ideal we can aspire towards.

Many parents will request a Vedic horoscope for the newborn, to help them understand more about their child's nature and its future. Vedic astrology is different from Western astrology in that it focuses on a person's inner nature, rather than on their outward personality. In *Autobiography of a Yogi,* Yogananda's teacher, Sri Yukteswar, explains that children waiting to be born pick their own time of birth in mathematical accordance with their own karma. Afterwards, he warns that the natal "horoscope is a challenging portrait, revealing [an] unalterable past and its probable future results," and that it "can be rightly interpreted only by [those few with] intuitive wisdom."*

A Vedic chart is a roadmap, not a rigid course to be followed without using one's own inner guidance. We have found that Vedic astrology is very helpful; every five years or so Nakula and I return for updates. Many consult

---

* Paramhansa Yogananda, *Autobiography of a Yogi* (Nevada City, California: Crystal Clarity Publishers, 2005), 163.

this tool in order to find auspicious times to hold a wedding or baptism ceremony, build a house or launch a new venture, start a career or choose a suitable life partner.

Hinduism has many birth rituals. For instance, before a child is born parents perform a special prayer, given as part of their obligation to continue the human race. There are prayers before conception, one of which is that a man, before relations with his wife, faces eastward and asks a blessing. During the third or fourth month of pregnancy a prayer for the fetus protection is performed to invoke divine qualities into the soul. These rituals are both wholesome and beautiful, and for some of them, a look at the deeper meanings can be helpful.

For instance, in the fourth or seventh months of pregnancy, the soon-to-be father combs his wife's hair, expressing his love and support for her. While this may seem frivolous, I can remember feeling fat and uncomfortable during the last months of my pregnancy. This simple and somewhat intimate ritual seems very appealing as a way for a husband to say, "I love your soul and the soul of our unborn child, and I will be there for both of you with all my love and devotion." It is another way for a husband to express to his wife, "God in me honors the God in you."

Baby showers are often held during the seventh month of pregnancy, and fire ceremonies are offered as a ritual to soothe expectant mothers. Some say that light instrumental music played at this time will refine the development of a baby's ears and sense of hearing.

Consider the music your unborn child may hear. During the sixth month of my pregnancy I sang with the choir many inspiring songs based on the life of Christ that my teacher had composed. The choir director had me stand right in the front row, and I had many rehearsals with him during my pregnancy. A few months after our son's birth, the director visited our home. As he walked in the door and started speaking, our son raised his arm, then smiled and made noises at him, as if welcoming an old friend. The two of them interacted quite naturally and we all commented on the fact that our time together in the choir was something our son was happy to remember.

The journey that parents take with their children offers many opportunities for yogis to accelerate spiritually. In the later part of the first stage of yoga, a child's path to independence can be most exciting, and also the most dangerous period of their life. There can be uncertainty and doubts, overconfidence, rebellion, and even pride.

In the peculiar twists of karma, many young people choose a different spiritual path rather than inheriting one from their kin. Yet the lessons of youth are foundations for a lifetime. How parents, friends, and family contribute to the myriad situations that surround each soul on their journey towards adulthood will either support or undermine their childrens' future.

CHAPTER 3

How Toddlers Teach Us

THE ROAD TO THE nursery school follows a steep ridge at the western boundary of the village. At the top of that hill, a panoramic view is favored by sunset watchers. In the evenings, star watchers come here to observe the heavens as we spin through space. The interconnectedness of our little lives can be felt in expansive vistas. From one side of the ridge, the view looks down onto rolling hills and valleys of the Sierra Nevada foothills. To the east, the hills climb upwards towards the snowcapped mountains of the High Sierra north of Lake Tahoe.

It was afternoon and time to pick up Rama from his preschool sojourn. By car, the approach up the ridge featured a steep rise that ended right near the door of the nursery school classroom. I parked our aging Honda sedan, pulled the emergency brake, stepped out of the car, and headed to the classroom.

Rama's teacher was a caring elder who doted over the children meticulously. After play sessions, she sometimes offered input and advice on everything from peer psychology to the latest homeopathic remedies. Today was one of those days, and I could sense she wanted to engage me. Normally, I would have collected our son quickly, as I'd learned he could get away from me quite easily. His teacher wanted to talk, and even now I wonder whether it was my need or hers that led me to spend those few extra minutes listening.

Parents have an inborn radar that tells them where their child is. Even though physically separate, there is this intuitive knowing that a part of you is somewhere else, running through the fields, or hanging upside down from a tree branch—or any number of worries meant to test our detachment and realization of the natural order of the universe. In yoga, our first step towards a broader understanding of interconnectedness starts with our closest relationships: for householders, it often begins with our children.

I was torn. This teacher needed someone to listen to her—and it was not that she wanted to share some trivial event related to children, their peer group, or nutritional choices. As my mind and heart focused on her words, I became oblivious to the classroom, the children, even my son.

After several minutes, my head turned. Where had Rama gone? I looked around the classroom; he was not there. My heart began to beat faster. Looking outside, I saw our old Honda slowly rolling backward as it inched down the ridge towards what I knew was an even steeper drop where the wheels would be fully spinning. My mind called to Babaji, the deathless guru from *Autobiography of a Yogi*. I believe I screamed Babaji's name as I ran out of the preschool, somehow thinking I could catch and halt the progress of the two tons of steel barreling down the hill before me.

I caught a glimpse of Rama at the helm, standing calmly between the driver's and the passenger seat, his hands on the dashboard looking just like a captain unaware of the rogue wave about to hit him. There was nothing that could stop him, and I could not catch him. My eyes shot to the long slope down the hill behind him and wondered how the crash might occur. My focus returned to Babaji. Within seconds, the car, which had been moving straight backwards, began to turn in a sharp angle and head towards an even steeper drop of the ridge that would insure a much quicker demise. I surrendered and watched in horror. Then it stopped. The bottom of the car had miraculously caught on a rock rising about fifteen inches from the ground. It was the only rock on that part of the ridge. The car was teetering there, and as I quickly rushed to the door, panic set in. If Rama moved or if I opened the door, would the car suddenly slide off its perch and take us both down the cliff? The fear on my face and the precarious position of the car were churning the ether.

Moments later, a car drove up and an elderly gentleman with white hair and wise eyes assessed the situation. His eyes locked with mine as if to say, *Don't move, I'll be right there.* He quickly parked his car, strode up, and calmly asked me for my keys, as though the situation was completely normal. Then he did what I could not do. He opened the door to my car, stepped inside, and quickly started it. With the car dipping up and down like a teeter-totter, and its wheels spinning furiously, he somehow drove it off the precipice and onto flat land.

I was trembling, and the combination of fear and relief that poured through my body was countered by deep gratitude to my friend. *How did that happen?* I felt a mixture of bewilderment and humility that my sincere call for help had been answered. Years later, whenever other accidents and challenging events occurred, I would go deep into my inner spine and respond to matters from that place of deep calmness.

A year earlier, when he was barely three, we took Rama on his first trip to a shopping mall. He was dressed in an adorable black-and-white striped jumpsuit, sort of like the kind a prisoner might wear, except this one had a cute little animal embroidered on its chest.

We were all eyeing the sales racks when Rama disappeared under a circular rack close to the floor. He quickly found that he could easily escape us and even outrun us. The race was on. We caught a glimpse of him as he zipped out the entrance to the department store and headed down the mall. Now we were all running.

This was our first venture, with our toddler, from country living into the jungle of the city, and we hadn't been prepared for his reaction. As we chased after him, I glimpsed him running in and out of stores at breakneck pace. My husband, aghast at the sudden stark reality of parenthood, began to call his name. Rama was long gone, his adorable playsuit a miasma of black and white amidst the horizon of shoppers. Thoughts of child abduction rose in my mind. Of course, anyone thinking along those lines would quickly reexamine their motives once they tried to restrain our son, let alone put him in a car seat.

After a twenty-minute chase, we finally caught Rama in a shoe store. I harbored a newfound gratitude and increased respect for my parents, who had raised seven of us children, not to mention two cousins that lived with us part time.

Child curiosity is a normal and intelligent response for children, and a child's energy level can quickly test even the most attentive parent. Finding creative ways to help channel their energy can be a challenge. I embarked on ways to engage my energetic son that didn't involve plopping him in front of a computer or a television screen.

Fresh air walks in the stroller, watching real life tractors and big machines operate, picking up sticks and rocks in the nearby forest, bouncing on the trampoline, creating an indoor fort with blankets and cardboard, encountering lizards, frogs, bugs, and anything that was in the territory of our own house or nearby became a cause for discovery. We painted, drew, read, and went on adventures. Nakula and I enjoy gardening, so we created a large vegetable kingdom behind our house. There was always plenty to do in the garden. We gave it lots of energy and it helped sustain us.

At one time the householder stage seemed full of career and work, meetings with clients, endless planning, making money, and looking for ways to get established in the world. Now, helping a youngster take a nap became the biggest focus of the day.

My friend Laura made use of the numerous hours she spent walking her son in a stroller as an opportunity to memorize the poem "Samadhi" composed by Yogananda to describe the highest state of consciousness. With the words written out on three-by-five cards, she repeated the poem again and again until it was emblazoned in her mind. It took many stroller rides, but now, twenty-seven years later, the poem remains with her.

The subtle energy of everything we do when we're with our little ones transfers easily to their consciousness. Holding your toddler and walking around a small room while chanting the most sacred of all Vedic mantras, the Gayatri mantra, is a great blessing for parent and child.

As parents, we can give children positive experiences that nullify messages of societal ills. We do this through our own intelligent choices, through prayers for our children and others, by getting outside and experiencing nature in a deeper way, through our daily spiritual practices, but mostly through our own healing love, energy and focus directed towards our children and each other.

Many of the parents in our yoga community have done their best to prevent video games from becoming an addictive force in our children's lives. Some of us went without television; and as we were somewhat remote, we had little exposure to mass media. For years, my son's only video exposure was an occasional episode of Barney the dinosaur, Mister Rogers' Neighborhood, or the talking puppet "Lamb Chop."

Nakula had a job that required him to commute to the city for several hours each day. During this time, to keep his mind uplifted and focused, he would play tapes of Swami Kriyananda chanting Sanskrit mantras. As Nakula was about to depart for work one morning, Rama was watching his weekly episode of the friendly lamb puppet singing the closing chorus of "This is the song that never ends, and it goes on and on my friend. . . .". Nakula exploded: "Can we not listen to that song anymore? It's beginning to enter my consciousness!" He explained that now, instead of the Gayatri mantra, all he could think of was Lamb Chop and "the song that never ends." We had a good laugh about it, but it was an important lesson.

If that song was affecting Nakula, how much more was it affecting Rama—or any child going through their early years without an adult's ability to filter what they hear?

CHAPTER 4

Yogic Schools for Youth

YOGA MEDITATION IS A science, not a religion. It can be employed by people of all belief systems to deepen their own faith and enrich their life experiences. Those who recognize what meditation can offer youth naturally hope it will someday be available in all schools. Research has shown its benefits, and schools worldwide are beginning to incorporate it into their curricula. With regular meditation students gain calmness, focus, and peace, achieve greater success, and learn to reduce stress in a natural way.

In America, pioneering efforts to bring yoga and meditation to schools began in 1972 at the Living Wisdom Schools located at Ananda Village in Northern California. The schools were founded with the belief that students need inspiration and training for life, in addition to preparation for employment and intellectual pursuits.

In 1975 the Maharishi School in Iowa began, based on the teachings of Maharishi Mahesh Yogi, founder of Transcendental Meditation. Today the school offers training from pre-school through PhD programs. Besides meditation, the Maharishi formulated the Science of Creative Intelligence (SCI), a systematic study of the laws of nature that underlie the structure and functioning of our world. He further designed how SCI could be used at any grade level, so that any subject can be connected to the knowledge of natural law, and to one's own self. In 2011, television celebrity host Oprah Winfrey visited the Maharishi schools and told the director, "I always wanted to help create an Age of Enlightenment, but I didn't know how."

Both the Living Wisdom Schools and the Maharishi schools have incorporated meditation into Western education for youth—as has the Mount Madonna School, which was founded in 1979 by Baba Haridas near Santa Cruz, California. In India the Miri Piri School in Amritsar, which Western students attend, was started by Yogi Bhajan. Likewise, many Indian teachers such as Anandamayi Ma, Amma, Sri Aurobindo, Sai Baba, and those from the Sivananda lineage have set up schools in India.

Though not founded on yogic and Vedic principles, other institutes of learning, like Rudolf Steiner's Waldorf Schools, (which first began in Germany in 1919), and Dr. Maria Montessori's Schools (which began in Italy), have brought holistic, child-centered education to the fore.

Studies from Harvard several years ago indicated that some of the most successful K–12 students were those who were home-schooled or in holistic programs offering smaller student-teacher ratios. In addition, research has long shown that parental involvement with children's education has produced lasting successful results.

In the summer of 2017 I spoke with Narani Moorhouse, who has taught in the Living Wisdom Schools for more than forty years and is the author of *Supporting Your Child's Inner Life*. I wanted to ask about discoveries she's made, while teaching in the past twenty years since she wrote her groundbreaking book. The Living Wisdom School has established innovative new teaching methods for academics and meditation. Narani has taught preschool through fifth grade, though her area of expertise is with young children.

"Children learn differently than adults," she said. "They need to experience something before they can understand it. They learn through movement, games, play, and stories." The curriculum she and others have developed is creative and profound.

I observed her with a group of yoga and meditation teachers at The Expanding Light training center at Ananda Village. She was teaching methods to help children meditate, concentrate, focus, and even attune to subtle realities. There were exercises with evocative names like "still as a stone" and "elevator breathing," plus a feather-breathing demonstration that taught young children breath control. "A child's lungs are very tiny," she explained. "As teachers we need to attune to our students. When an exercise is finished, instead of asking the children how they liked it, we watch their faces. We've learned not to talk too much—children live in the heart, not in the mind."

Narani told me that the Living Wisdom Schools were shifting how they assess various qualities they are teaching children. "For instance," she said, "math requires clarity of thinking." Now, instead of just teaching math in the standard way, the school is instead finding new means to teach clarity of thinking that also involves math. "We're looking at how we can more effectively teach the specific qualities that help children become more successful in life," she added.

The Living Wisdom Schools are based on a unique academic curriculum that stresses nonsectarian values and ethics carefully designed to meet each individual's need, to prepare students for life's inner and outer challenges, and to encourage a rich, lifelong journey of adventure and self-discovery. In 1986 the community founder, Swami Kriyananda, wrote *Education for Life*. In that book he describes four stages of learning associated with various age groups of children. These stages include the foundation years, the feeling years, the willful years, and the thoughtful years. From this book, the Education for Life (EFL) foundation was created to train and support teachers and schools with new methods for helping children and young adults become successful in the fullest sense of the word.

The stresses caused by societal ills, academic pressure, peer pressure, and a focus on wealth and power are some of the most challenging aspects of a young person's life. Children begin life protected and supported by loving parents, only to discover that society and traditional education are geared to steer them towards becoming high achievers. Likewise, nurturing home and school environments are often at odds with the heavy emphasis in today's culture on substance abuse, sex, and violence.

At Ananda, middle and high school students gain confidence through direct experiences set up to help them succeed. They need (and are encouraged) to ask questions and form their own conclusions. In this process they receive support from teachers to explore ideas.

I spoke with Gary McSweeney, a teacher in the Living Wisdom Middle School in Palo Alto. What did the school do to help preteens and young teens, besides offering yoga postures?

"Once, a group of middle school students took a field trip to watch the sunset at Half Moon Bay, while another teacher and I prepared dinner. Not a lot was said when they returned, but over the next few months, through their writing, we realized that several of them had had transcendent experiences—unique to each one. Hard to put into words, but they had experienced something beyond the usual."

"What was that, exactly?" I asked him.

"Perhaps it was a sense of belonging, or purpose, direction, connection. I prefer to witness the change and take note without digging into the specifics, because I feel those are between the student and God, or spirit. Whether you use the word "God" or something else, these students have undergone experiences of clarity and depth, belonging to something larger, and received a context for life, and hope."

I asked him about the philosophy of the school. "We are nontraditional. Our school culture is based on caring and compassion. We have a unique system here for conflict resolution that we've developed over more than twenty-five years," he said. "We don't offer letter grades: there are no standardized tests. We take morning walks together, do energizing exercises, meditate, and offer healing prayers."

"Each year we put on a play about a great saint from one of the world's wisdom traditions. This process goes on for six weeks. We start thinking about our performance in September; but we talk about it all year, both before and after the actual event. Students do research papers on the people we study. We rehearse for two hours at a stretch, and we schedule four performances for the local Bay Area communities," he explained.

"Atheists have visited our school and afterward reported that we're not dogmatic; we're nonsectarian, experiential. We're not espousing any particular Eastern or Western religion. The closest philosophy to ours is 'Sanaatan

Dharma,' which, even though it has its roots in Hinduism, is based on the deeper teachings of yoga. We see the truth underlying all religions. We focus on qualities, not dogmas. For instance, students learn that when they're kind to others, they themselves become happier.

"To me, teaching is akin to being a life coach. I've worked in summer camps and I've always enjoyed working with youths. Teaching in this school requires me to use my intuition, derived from years of daily meditation.

"In working with the students, I use humor and laughter, suggest boundaries, encourage and cajole, and model mature behavior. We use happiness and patience as a guide. I've learned to tune in to these students. You may think that you know a lot, but we teachers learn from observing the youth.

"How do you develop intuition? By sitting in silence at the end of your meditation, after practicing your mantra and other techniques. Intuition, creativity, these come from meditation—and I apply them to teaching science or any other subject—or really, everything I do."

For several years the nearby high schools in Palo Alto have experienced the heartache of cluster suicides. I was curious how Gary's school helped students avoid these tragedies.

"We're different because we emphasize the positive and the highest potential in each student. We don't focus as much on intellectual competition; and it's already intensely competitive here in Silicon Valley. When a school's focus is all about getting straight A's, students can become mean, selfish, and unhappy," he said. "The youth that come here grow up to be happier, so we ask parents, 'Do they trust their hearts, or do they trust their minds?'"

"Can you offer an example?" I asked.

He replied, "I've had parents tell me, 'You saved my daughter's life.'"

"One of our challenges is conveying to parents the universal spirituality that our school works to instill in its students. Many people believe that 'My religion is the best.' We familiarize middle-schoolers with modern mystics like Thoreau, Emerson, George Washington Carver, and Dr. Martin Luther King."

The teachings of yoga are beneficial for people of all ages. In a physical sense, yoga and meditation keep the body and mind lubricated and flexible. When the mind and body are flexible, people adapt easier. Some of today's educational systems are falling short in meeting teenagers' needs. Studies have found that the suicide rate for teenage girls in America is up by 40 percent. Teen depression is also on the rise. Today in Palo Alto, right near Stanford University, the Living Wisdom High School, where Gary McSweeney teaches, offers a strikingly different approach to education.

According to the *Palo Alto Weekly*, "Students applying are asked not about grades or test scores but to describe the qualities they like most about themselves and admire in others. A grid titled 'How do you see yourself?' asks prospective students to evaluate themselves on qualities like willpower, curiosity, open mindedness, and personal happiness." The article goes on to say that the curriculum includes daily meditation, adventure, and self-discovery, in addition to academic rigor.

Recent research indicates that after high school and college, young people may need more time to become established. Emerging neuroscience suggests that most brains aren't fully developed until the age of twenty-five. Many times I have worked with young adults who, after four years of college, have changed their minds and are no longer interested in the degree focus they had committed to. There are alternatives now that allow young people to discover their natural life-work and talents, and to help them realize a success that is measured not in terms of outward conditioning but inner happiness.

Unfortunately, in mainstream public education, the bureaucratic systems of standardized testing and assembly-line learning have made it challenging and inconvenient to adapt to more individualized learning. When bureaucracy rules an organization, rigidity can lead to less creativity and openness to new ideas.

It used to be a standing joke that when potential students and parents arrive at our Ananda College campus, (located in a remote forest), the first thing they would ask was, "Where's the college?" We are conditioned by society to view form as being a precursor to wisdom. The great quantum theoretical physicist Amit Goswami, author of *The Self-Aware Universe*, first visited our college when it was located at the rural meditation retreat where our family lives. (Goswami starred in the popular *What the Bleep Do We Know!?* documentary, and some have compared him to Einstein.)

After he stepped out of the car and walked around the retreat campus for a few minutes, he exclaimed, "Wow, the energy here is amazing!" Later, he congratulated our students for learning what he called "non-local communication" through our practice of meditating together in groups.

Because energy is subtle and non-linear, the results of meditation help in unimaginable ways. What Dr. Goswami was seeing in our college was not its outward form, but the underlying energy. Our college is nontraditional, and even today we're small enough that we can change the way we function to adapt to the future.*

I mentioned earlier that, according to Yogananda's guru, Sri Yukteswar, and ancient Vedic teachings, our planet has recently entered the Age of Energy. Some colleges of the future will be focused on energy, not form. They'll teach subjects like the science of attunement, magnetism, quantum physics, energy healing, world cultures and consciousness, yoga therapy, alternative education, the arts as a vehicle for higher consciousness, and mastery over oneself through the study of Self-realization.

As scientists learn more about subtle energy, their pursuits will bring them more in touch with the realm of spirit. And it may be that someday universities will teach such esoteric subjects as bilocation—the ability to manifest the physical body in two locations simultaneously—an advanced spiritual power that a number of great yogis have demonstrated throughout history.

---

* Teachers can receive online and residential training in Education for Life (EFL) for preschool through twelfth grade. There are Living Wisdom campuses in Seattle; Palo Alto; Portland, Oregon; Assisi, Italy; and in Slovenia. There is also a Living Wisdom High School at Ananda Village in Nevada City, California, which includes a boarding school for young adults. The school was founded in 2000, has WASC accreditation, and offers college prep-style classes—as well as the EFL techniques that mirror Yogananda's ideals for balanced living. Young adults can attend internship programs at Ananda Village. In addition, the Ananda University currently offers online programs.

CHAPTER 5

Girls' Rites

"The White Buffalo Woman spoke to the women, telling them that
it was the work of their hands and the fruit of their bodies which
kept the people alive. 'You are from the mother earth,' she told
them. 'What you are doing is as great as what warriors do.'"
—Native American wisdom

THE TRAIL TO BALD Mountain is as gnarled as the Manzanita that engulfs it. At the end lies a steep lookout rock. I had climbed halfway up the rock when a large eagle soared into view, about twenty feet above. Hiking with a friend, we must have startled it. It began to swirl higher and higher, disappearing into the stratosphere. I'd never seen a bird ascend so quickly.

Eagles are sacred to Native American traditions for flying the highest, observing the earth in all directions, and offering the gifts of perception and illumination. Some traditions teach how to "become" the eagle, a symbolism for heroism, nobility, and spirituality. The lookout rock of Bald Mountain was considered a holy area by Native Americans who inhabited this part of Northern California hundreds of years ago.

Bald Mountain offers a 360-degree view of the area. Below it is a thousand-foot drop to the South Yuba River Gorge. Standing on the rock, one can see east to the snow-capped High Sierras. To the south, beyond the foothills, lies the Sacramento Valley. To the west lie more foothills and another sacred Native American mountain. To the northwest and six miles away is Ananda Village. And directly north is the Ananda Meditation Retreat. The influences of all four directions can be seen and felt at this spot.

An Indian stone circle, used for sacred ceremonies, remains near the lookout rock. One can almost imagine what it might have been like, centuries ago, in this very spot. A clear night would be spent deciphering the stars above. A roaring fire in the middle of the circle would keep warmth for ceremonies. There might be storytelling, dancing, or drumming, with perhaps a spiritual elder offering healing chants to a small group of youth.

On a clear day, if one is walking southwest towards the beginning of the Bald Mountain trail, the Sutter Buttes can be seen on the far westerly horizon. They rise like a camel's spine, an ascending island amid the flat Sacramento Valley. According to some legends, the Sutter Buttes are "Spirit Mountains": a way station where the spirits of the Native Americans rested before their journey to the afterlife. Some consider these mountains a power spot reserved for healers and spiritual leaders.

Bald Mountain is about a thirty-minute hike from the Ananda Meditation Retreat, where I live. For the past fifty years, the retreat has been a place where people gather for seclusion, renewal, and healing. In 1967, when Swami Kriyananda first walked this land, he felt it had already been blessed as holy ground. He and three others—a Roshi from the San Francisco Zen Community, and poets Gary Snyder and Allan Ginsberg—each purchased land here to create retreats.

Our neighbor Gary Snyder, author of *Turtle Island,* told us that the McNab Cypress, a tree that grows in few parts of the world, has a small foothold near Bald Mountain. He also said he thought the very land where the retreat stands had once been a Native American acorn orchard. "This is the highest altitude these types of oaks grow," he explained. Once, while speaking to our college students, Gary told the history of this place, a moving account of what historians and geologists report existed here hundreds and thousands of years ago. Now eighty-seven, Gary is considered a wise elder for many environmentalists, championing the earth at a time when it needs it.

A tangible sense of peace surrounds the meditation retreat and the nearby forests. While leading a poetry class under a tunnel of Manzanita trees, we began our writing with a meditation, attuning to the Native Americans. Nature and silence are ideal for inward reflection, especially for the youth.

In many cultures, when a young girl begins to exhibit physical signs of puberty, it can be a sign that other things may be developing as well. Each child is unique, but around the age of eleven or twelve, a girl experiences her first menses; though menstrual cycles can start anytime between the ages of eight and sixteen. From eleven to fourteen, girls are entering their "will" years. Their bodies may be changing, they may be experiencing new emotions, and their hormone levels may also be increasing. Awkwardness, self-consciousness, and a newfound timidity or rebelliousness may occur.

In some Native American traditions, celebrating the first menses is ideal for a rite of passage, helping girls acknowledge their transition towards adulthood. When an educator asked me about vision quests and rites of passage for thirteen- to fourteen-year-old girls, I remembered what Swami Kriyananda had said to me during an interview with him in 1998. "Draw from the Native American culture for rites of passage. They have beautiful ceremonies."

I meditated on his words. He had not said to *duplicate* the ceremonies but to *draw from* them. We needed to attune to the inherent wisdom the Native American ceremonies acknowledged in young people. Native American culture honors the earth and the natural environment in a manner similar to Vedic and yogic philosophy. Specifically, the power of the natural world to communicate with us offers many layers of symbolism and awareness for youths.

The Ananda Meditation Retreat encompasses seventy acres of woodland meadows and forests. The retreat is far from civilization, surrounded on all sides by over four thousand acres of Bureau of Land Management (BLM) forests, and adjacent to the old-growth 'Inimim Forest. ('Inimim is the Nisenan word for ponderosa pine.) The Nisenan are the indigenous people that lived in this area. The area is home to California black bears, deer, foxes, bobcats, mountain lions, coyotes, squirrels, and a variety of woodpeckers, birds, and other sentient beings. All these can be a part of a story or vision that comes to a young girl on a sacred quest. Native American animal symbolism is one way the spirit world sends us messages. In a landscape void of humans, all life becomes conversation. Through solitude and attunement comes deeper awareness.

Naturalist and author Joseph Cornell, a yogi who once lived at the Meditation Retreat for many years, explains how to conduct an "Interview with Nature": an exercise he included in his book *Sharing Nature*. "Wild animals and plants attract us because we have a natural affinity for those sharing the gift of life. Humanizing nature helps us feel to some degree that all beings are like us," he writes. Cornell's powerful Interview with Nature exercise can be done by children, teens, or adults. The interviewer must attune to the rock, plant, tree, or natural feature. The observer learns as much as possible about the subject, asking silent questions to tune in to its point of view. With this idea in mind, we began to formulate the preparation for a vision quest in sacred nature.

During the period of a few months, I enjoyed several conversations with an Italian teacher very familiar with Native American customs and rites of passage. We were brainstorming cycles-of-life ceremonies for a particular group of girls in the Living Wisdom Schools. We decided accommodating a large group of girls would be difficult. With a small group of four to eight girls, however, there would be less peer pressure. Youths learn from their peers. They watch what others are doing and naturally want to fit in and feel comfortable.

Our goal was to spend the entire day in silence using the grounds and nearby forests of the Meditation Retreat. In the morning the girls did yoga postures and performed various ceremonies, then hiked in silence to Bald Mountain and the sacred Indian circle. Native American activities were incorporated into the day.

The vision quest is the most well-known rite of passage common to Native American traditions. Author Jamie Sams is part Cherokee and Seneca. She once mentioned an experience she had in a traditional four-day quest where she fasted and prayed in an effort to invoke a vision that would help her gain direction in life. Around midnight on the third night of her vision quest, she saw stars in the sky turning many different colors, even singing to her. Through this experience Jamie Sams gained her Medicine name, Midnight Song.

With deep respect honoring the Native American tradition and the principles it represents, we created a transformative experience that incorporated Vedic and yogic traditions as well. We would begin the ceremony at a small earthen hand-built cob temple the Ananda College students had helped construct, located on the Meditation Retreat campus.

The highlight of the day was the three to four hours each girl spent alone in nature, far away from the possibility of human interaction. The forest provided a wild landscape where the girls would each look for their own power place. Once they located their sacred spot, they would cordon it off, creating a wide circle of at least ten feet around them. The circle would be marked with cornmeal, a grain favored by Native Americans. They would stay there for three hours. During their time alone, they would seek a vision or insight, something that would help them to achieve the highest within themselves. There were no restrictions as to what they could do in the circle—dance, chant, sing, meditate, pray—anything that would not distract them from their true purpose. They realized that if they were to attract a spirit animal or bird, they would need to spend time in inner stillness and silence.

When the teachers discussed journaling, or creating something in the circle, we felt this would distract the girls from the higher purpose of receiving a vision. Afterwards, if a living entity didn't appear to them, a vision or dream might come to them a few days later. Sometimes this happens after the actual vision quest. Encouraging youths to journal or create art about their experience a few days or a week afterwards is one way to follow-up the quest. Likewise, it's helpful not to give too much information before the vision quest, so the youths wouldn't be stimulated to draw something from their imagination. By clearing their minds and focusing through meditation they would draw an authentic experience that would serve as a symbol for their next step in life.

The book *Animal Speak* by Ted Andrews is a wonderful dictionary of the Native American interpretations of the symbolic meanings of hundreds of animals, birds, and plants. I received a copy many years ago from a shaman who is also an intuitive. To a yogi, the depth of connection to all life is unspoken knowledge. Subtle clues, such as how a living creature appears, when it appears, which direction it moves, can all serve as communication.

After the vision quest the girls spent two hours in silence with follow-up projects and more time for yoga postures and meditation. Before dinner, the girls and their leaders joined me in the retreat kitchen to prepare the meal. We began by lighting a candle and repeating a prayer in front of a small kitchen altar. "Divine Mother, come into our hearts and into our hands, that the food we prepare for others be holy." We then chanted the sacred Sanskrit word Om three times to bless the kitchen and our dinner preparations.

Giggles erupted when I mentioned the girls would prepare food together in total silence. Teenage girls love to have fun, and it's easy to get distracted by little conversations and diversions. It was my task to model calmness and centeredness. When the entire focus is given to preparing food, especially in silence, it becomes its own ceremony. The concept of preparing food in a sacred manner is not new. Many cultures believe that the vibrations that go into food while cooking can enhance it and offer healing on subtle levels. On this particular evening, the girls served the food on a buffet table set for guests. We sang a prayer together with the retreat guests to bless the food once more. "Receive Lord, in Thy Light, the food we eat for it is Thine. Infuse it with Thy love, Thy energy, Thy life divine."

During the meal the girls attempted to sit in silence, maintaining the spiritual momentum they had created that day. According to yogic and Ayurveda principles, mindful eating in silence is good for the digestion, and allows the vibrations put into the food to be absorbed in a more conscious way. For many years, when the college ran the retreat, the cooks would post signs that read "Kitchen in Silence" so that anyone entering would know that the equivalent of a sacred ceremony was in process. Over the years we learned and utilized Sanskrit blessings, Buddhist prayers, Christian, Jewish, and Sufi prayers, and Yogananda's prayer before eating.

In my experience, a meaningful ritual for young people is learning how to chant mantras.

One evening when I was a young woman living in the Bay Area, I had an interesting encounter with people I feared might hurt me. I was walking through an underground tunnel, filled with gang members and graffiti. As I began to panic, a mantra I'd never heard before came into my head.

"Om Namo Bhagavate Vasudevaya." I repeated this unfamiliar mantra until I arrived safely on the other side. Many years later I discovered what the mantra meant. A rough translation is: "Abandon all concern with religious prescriptions and dogmas and simply surrender to Me. I will deliver you from all sin. Do not fear." This mantra is also meant to invoke the blessings of Lord Krishna, and it is the primary mantra extolled by India's "Bible," the Bhagavad Gita.

After dinner we met at the retreat area used for Vedic fire ceremonies, a large circle with benches surrounding it. I shared the reasoning behind the fire ceremony and mantras.

We were using the exact location where my teacher had performed daily fire ceremonies fifty years previous. We still use these mantras in ceremonies at the yoga community.

The Vedic fire ceremony was the culmination of an inward day for the girls. The mantras are a powerful oral tradition used for thousands, perhaps millions of years by the rishis and higher civilizations of Vedic India. Their sounds and intonations are very important, and for this reason they should be chanted correctly, lest their subtle meaning become lost. While I have studied and used these mantras for more than thirty years, I find their energy ever-new and revealing.

The girls created a small bonfire, made with kindling they had gathered, and helped to replenish the flames as needed. The girls took part in the ceremony. While performing the Gayatri Mantra, a teaspoon of ghee, or clarified butter, is poured into the fire at the end of each recitation. (The ghee is a symbol of one's pure aspirations, to be transformed by the fire and through the mantras.) When we did the second, Mahamritunjaya Mantra, everyone took a small handful of rice, and, at the end of each repetition, offered a few grains into the fire. (The rice is a symbol of the seeds of karma to be burned up and purified in the sacred light of the fire.)

The light from a Vedic fire ceremony symbolizes the purifying and burning away of those habits and attachments that keep us from inner happiness. Though life appears to be constantly changing, the power of the mantras reflect the still, unchanging depth of spirit that connects us all.

The first mantra we chanted is considered the most sacred in Vedic India and yoga ashrams. Often in India the Gayatri Mantra is chanted at sunrise, a prayer offered before the dawn, or at the beginning of a sacred ceremony. It is a mantra for enlightenment, a prayer for the realization of supreme truths, a calling on the Divine. A general translation of the Gayatri Mantra is "We meditate upon the Supreme Light of the three (the physical, energetic or 'astral,' and mental or 'causal') universes. May it enlighten our consciousness."

Gayatri Mantra:
Oṃ bhūr bhuvaḥ swaḥa
Om tát savitúr váreṇiyaṃ
bhárgo devásya dhīmahi
dhíyo yó naḥa prachodáyāt, Om.

We chanted the mantra an auspicious number of times, invoking its intent, and offering ghee into the fire after each incantation, as a means of purifying our intentions and prayers. During longer ceremonies we may chant each mantra 108 times. The second, Mahamritunjaya Mantra, is considered ideal for spiritual liberation. It bestows longevity, and is designed to cure illness. It is said to ward off negative forces by creating a protective psychic shield around the practitioner. The general translation for this mantra is: "We worship the Omniscient One Who nourishes all living beings. May He free us from death and grant us immortality."

The Mahamitrunjaya Mantra is also associated with Shiva. An ideal time to recite it is at dusk or during the evening.

Mahamitrunjaya Mantra:
Om tryambakam yajaamahey
sugandhim pushthi vardhanam;
Urvaa rukameya bandhanaan
Mrityor muksheeya maamritaat. Om.*

---

* The *Mantra* CD from Crystal Clarity Publishers contains chanting of both the Gayatri and Mahamritunjaya mantras, so that you can follow along and over time learn them. This CD is available by visiting crystalclarity.com/shop/music/mantra/

The Vedic mantras contain layers of subtle meaning instilled by the rishis. The rishis were seers and saints who developed these mantras at a time when the consciousness of the planet was much higher and more evolved. Today, groups like Euphonic Yoga in India are incorporating mantras and sounds of the chakras with instrumental music, hand mudras (gestures), and yogic dance movements that uplift and energize. Scientists are just beginning to understand subtle energy, sound rhythm, and their role in healing, yet the Vedic culture has always been aware of them.

Following a day of vision quest and the celebration dinner, the Vedic fire ceremony was capped off by the minutes we spent quietly enjoying the night air and the sacredness of the fire. Fire is a symbol in many cultures. While watching a fire burn, one can reflect on the mantras and attune to their power. The oral tradition of passing on sacred mantras, songs, and stories from one generation to the next is something today's youth can relate to.

Afterwards, as the fire burned down, the girls shared stories from their day. They didn't want to talk too much: a good sign. The evening culminated with a special blessing and each girl received a Native American token.

Five Step Process

First, the girls met in the small temple for yoga. Then, they hiked to Bald Mountain, and all the activities they did in the Native American Circle were designed to awaken the girls' enthusiasm. Third, they needed a place deep in nature—it could be a forest, a desert, or some other sacred place. Fourth, the girls attempted to fast, taking no food from breakfast until dinner, using only water. (This was surprisingly easy for them. If it had been difficult for any of them, they carried a few dried fruits and nuts to sustain them.) The fifth step was to share inspiration with their peers in the vision quest. (This is also something that could have been done around the fire at the close of the ceremony. In addition, during the weeks following the quest, some of the girls felt to share their experiences with other Living Wisdom High School students, teachers, and parents.)

At Ananda Village, a yogic afterschool group called "Spirit Warriors" offers many uplifting activities for younger girls age nine to twelve. Developing ceremonies and rites for girls can be an ongoing adventure.

CHAPTER 6

Boys' Rites

YOGANANDA ONCE TOLD HIS followers of a document, found in a Tibetan monastery, that chronicled the early life of Jesus—his lost years—which occurred between his twelfth and thirtieth years. During those lost years, which are not even mentioned in the gospels, Jesus conferred with the wise men of the East, who were from India. He learned from the wise men the mysteries of the inner life. Jesus was returning the visit they had paid him at his birth.

The tender years of a youth's journey into manhood can be a meaningful time. Rites of passage become influential when their spiritual significance is highlighted and enhanced.

A young man who grew up at Ananda Village had a unique rite of passage. I interviewed Simon for this book, and he was happy to share his story.

It is not unusual for young children to have fears of the unknown, fears drawn from their imagination, or even fears brought over from previous incarnations. When Simon was a toddler he was somewhat shy and fearful of being without his mother, and wasn't too keen on being left alone with a teacher, let alone other children. He needed to gently lessen the bonds with his mother so that he could begin attending kindergarten at the Ananda School. Knowing that Simon also had an adventurous side, his parents designed an event that would help him "graduate" from home to kindergarten.

Rising early one morning, his mother Laura began to prepare him for his rite-of-passage adventure.

It was still quite dark, the hum of crickets thick in the summer air. In the 1990s, a trail emerged in our yoga community from Maidu Ridge to Pubble Pond. Back then, the path felt more like a tunnel of underbrush and blackberry thickets, a place where wild animals might live. Mother and son walked the half-mile from their small cabin at Kailash Circle to the thicket trail. Leading Simon down the trail, Laura let him know that his father, Michael, and Narada, a close family friend, would meet him at the other end of the thicket, about five hundred feet away.

Once Simon appeared at the other end of the trail, the two older men led him down to Pubble Pond, where the three boarded a canoe. In the early dawn before sunrise, they all paddled in silence through the cool water, the older men whispering Sanskrit chants of courage. Candles were lit, a stick of incense was offered to the Divine, and sacred rose petals left over from a Kriya Yoga ceremony were showered on Simon. The chanting continued as they paddled together. After sunrise, the three returned to their cabin, where Laura had prepared a breakfast feast. Afterwards, Simon was presented with a bow for archery, a symbol of bravery.

When he was twenty-five, I asked Simon what that experience had been like for him—what he remembered of it, the impressions it left on him. "I had a lot of different fears back then. I was afraid of the dark, of shadows, of light shifting, of essentially being alone with the unknown. I was even afraid of Lotus Lane, a short driveway that was near my home. When you're five, the world seems much bigger and scarier." He admitted the bow he'd received for his bravery was a wonderful prize. "It was a compound bow, not a wimpy kid's bow," he said. After that experience, it was much easier for Simon to venture off to kindergarten, armed with newfound courage.

In a higher age, communities would partake in the prayers and good wishes for each young man going through their transition. Wise elders would offer words of encouragement. The youths would come before the elders for their blessings. Various members would offer their love, wisdom, and support.

Around the age of eleven (or even younger) is an ideal time to offer rites of passage for boys. To offer rites before their adolescence or when they are transitioning can be profound for a boy struggling with the concepts of manhood, and all the fears and questions it holds. In higher ages, and even in today's cultures, youth go off to live in a monastery or temple school to learn sacred ways of living.

In traditional Native American lore, a young boy's vision quest would occur near the time he reached puberty. Ideally, the quest should take place in solitude, in a natural surrounding with few distractions—like a forest, desert, or wilderness. During this quest is the time to ask, pray, or "cry out" for a vision that will help in one's life journey.

Before they embark on a vision quest, it's customary that Native American youths enter a sweat lodge where they would experience a preparatory cleansing and smudging ritual. After the sweat they would bathe in cold water. Next, the significance of the quest would be discussed with an elder, shaman, or priest. The youths would then go into isolation in the forest for three days and pray for their vision. Finally, they would meet with a shaman who would talk with them about their spirit animal and its importance in their new life as a young man. The event was concluded with a special ceremony and feast, and the young man might receive a special token, symbolic of the event.

Before many Native American vision quests one is encouraged to fast. The fasting is to help cleanse the body of toxins and offer deeper awareness, preparing a void within that spirit can fill. While many yogis also fast during seclusion, there are health challenges that need to be kept in mind before embarking on one.

One year a middle school held a modified rite of passage for young boys at the Meditation Retreat. The group spent time at the retreat in various inward activities before hiking down a very long and steep trail through the Yuba River Gorge to the South Yuba River, thousands of feet beneath the surrounding adjacent forests. The boys spent the night at a remote spot near the river, a place rarely frequented by humans.

There are mountain lions in this part of the Sierra Nevada. You never know when they are near; they are deft at tracking and hiding. In thirty years of living here I have never seen one. Even Satya, an elder who lived at the remote Ananda Meditation Retreat for forty-five years, never encountered the elusive cougar. Animals sense our fear. It is my belief that wild animals can sense the peace and calmness that resides within people, and will not approach humans unless provoked, or caring for their young.

According to some Native American traditions, animal totems or spirit guardians communicate the primordial consciousness. Even plant and tree spirits communicate in subtle ways. In Native American culture, the bear symbolizes awakening the power of the unconscious, or "wisdom coming to you," while the mountain lion symbolizes "coming into your own power."

For boys transitioning into young men, the importance of a rite of passage helps not only to validate the journey they are about to embark on, it gives them an inner badge of courage that will help them throughout their lives. There are other rites of passage for boys.

A group of Living Wisdom Junior High School boys traveled with one of their leaders from Northern California to Montana, to the headwaters of the Missouri River. Their goal was to canoe down the river, using the same path that Lewis and Clark had taken while discovering the West. "The land was barren and desolate," one of the youths recalled. "We were roughing it. We had to get up early, make a fire, make breakfast, get on the boats, and raft or paddle down the river. It wasn't easy." I asked if he had any outstanding memories from that trip.

"Every day the weather was different, so we were always on alert. One day I was riding at the rear of all the canoes with our leader. We had tied two canoes together into a makeshift catamaran that allowed us to carry all our gear. We were always the slowest rafters, far behind the others. On this particular day the weather changed dramatically. A squall came up and we were getting a tailwind. We decided to make a homemade sail using a tarp and a pole. Suddenly our catamaran was moving really fast, sailing past all the forward canoes—it was an amazing experience. On the last day of the trip it actually snowed while we were canoeing, which was a real challenge."

Each year the Living Wisdom High School teens take adventure trips. During these trips the youth are far away from things that have become familiar in their lives back home. On one trip the students volunteered in a turtle refuge area on an island off the eastern coast of Costa Rica. They counted turtle eggs, looked for nest disruption, and warded off potential poachers. "We had night duty watching for turtle poachers," one leader explained. "We'd split into groups of two and walk the beaches with flashlights, looking for the nests since that was when the turtles were active. We stayed at a rustic place where we ate beans and rice day in and day out, nothing else."

The leatherback sea turtles are endangered. Weighing up to fourteen hundred pounds and sporting a leathery soft shell designed to let them stay under water for longer periods of time, the survival of their eggs in the island beaches off Costa Rica has become a struggle between poachers and protectors. Allowing youths to be guardians of sea turtles offers a way to empower and engage their warrior qualities in a positive way. As all sea turtles lay their eggs on land, the turtle represents the transition from earth to water. In many Native American cultures, turtles represent Mother Earth and serve as a reminder that we live in a mutually beneficial existence—as we care for the earth, so she will care for and nurture us. For rites of passage, as we endeavor to draw from the wisdom of the Native American culture, we see that the philosophy of yoga has much in common with the understanding and communion that Native Americans and other indigenous tribes share with all life.

Those youths raised within the secure boundaries of a rural spiritual community required different challenges. I asked one former student what was the hardest thing he had to do when he was a teen. "It was the summer I spent in the city at an arts seminar when I was fifteen," he said. "I'd never lived around a lot of people or spent time in the city. I had to make all my own decisions, and I wasn't used to it. My initial response was to hide in my dorm room and go on Facebook. I grew up a lot because I was outside my comfort zone. I had to go out and meet people and make new friends, which was a new experience for me."

I once asked a Native American what his own sacred rite of passage had been like when he was a young boy. He had grown up on a reservation in the Southwest. "Back then, my father took me out into the wilderness and left me there. I fasted for four days and four nights. It was terrifying. I was scared of mountain lions. After my time alone, I finally had a vision, an experience I've never forgotten. The message was deeply personal for me, and it still has meaning for me to this day."

Now that he has a teenage son, I was curious if he intended to carry on a rite-of-passage tradition. "We live in the city now and it has a different set of dangers. Just as I had to be fearful of wild animals coming upon me, now I talk with my son about the dangers of gangs, drug dealers, and people who might harm him. I share with him how these people are looking for his weaknesses," he related. "We also talk about how he will navigate the obstacles of the city streets that call to him." He said he talks with his son about how gangs and drug dealers are like dangerous predators who could take his life and energy. He talked about the sacred bonds shared by father and son, and how he has to work to nurture those bonds.

When fathers and sons spend time together, every moment is meaningful. Even mundane chores like doing dishes, cutting wood, or cleaning a room offer silent opportunities. By allowing our sons and daughters to lead us in some activities, we model for them how to follow, and watch what happens.

The people of India consider it sacred to bathe in the Ganges, especially during a pilgrimage to the holy city of Rishikesh. Bathing in that river is believed to cleanse sins and bring liberation to the soul. On the surface, the river appears like sheets of glass meandering through the landscape. Yet the Ganges can swallow a life in seconds.

On one of our college trips to India, older high school students joined us. We were told by our hosts to be careful of the Ganges—an entire family had recently vanished under her waves. First, one member of the family waded too far out into the river, got caught, and drowned. Another family member rushed to lend a hand, and he got caught also. Then a young woman raced out to help him, and another, until five members of the same family were swept away and drowned over the course of a few minutes.

We were perched on a bank high above the Ganges when some of the students began jumping off a cliff into what appeared to be the shallow side of the volatile river. It seemed relatively safe until one of the older, stronger young men began to swim farther out into the river. With the memory of the disappearing family fresh in my mind, I ran to the water's edge and called to the younger student. The older student was already midway across the Ganges, swimming strongly. I quickly visualized them both surrounded in blue light, and offered prayers. I wasn't sure they'd make it across.

As the current strengthened, the younger student turned back and safely came ashore. The stronger swimmer continued through the most perilous part of the river. We were all watching and praying. We saw him slow down a bit, then continue on. It took a while for him to make the entire crossing, but he did. Then, as if to surprise us all, he exited the river onto the other side, walked up river a short distance, and swam back across to us.

Those of us watching this scene unfold were stunned. In retrospect, his swim across the Ganges, however frightening, felt like a rite of passage. It offered just the right degree of physical challenge and exercise of willpower for that particular young adult. Furthermore, it was spontaneous and unexpected, something that can't always be planned.

When co-creating rites of passage, it is helpful to consider environments that are challenging and out of one's comfort zone. The awareness and consciousness of the leaders or teachers is very important, as safety must be a primary concern. A leader who meditates, or has developed intuition and sensitivity to their students, can determine the circumstances that would offer a high rate of challenge, adventure, and personal transformation.

CHAPTER 7

Ingrid's Message

PARENTS FOLLOWING THE PATH of yoga can attract into their lives spiritually oriented children. An essential lesson for truth seekers is to recognize that the children they raise belong to the Infinite even more than to their own flesh and blood. This is often difficult to grasp when parents are in the throes of raising young children. The Divine, in a way that may seem impersonal to us, may have something else in mind for our children, and that intention may remain hidden for many years. Or, it can be evident from a young age, as it was in the case of Ingrid.

Ingrid is an intuitive who was born to spiritual parents. Her father was a meditating yogi. I chose to interview Ingrid for this book because I was aware that she could offer a perspective for young people and parents. The following is taken from that interview.

"I can remember my first channeling experience," Ingrid said. "It took place when I was seven years old. I'd had a low-grade fever and a man showed up in my head very clearly. He told me a story about fading away, and afterwards I wrote a poem from his perspective. The next day my dad complimented me on my poem. I was clairaudient and clairvoyant. At the time, I didn't know what was happening to me was not typical.

"I had regular visitations from light beings, and recognized at some point that I needed to spend a great deal of time alone. I was home-schooled. My father, as a yogi, started each day with yoga postures, chanting, and meditation.

But he also did something else. When we were meditating with our eyes shut, my dad put a compass in front of us, on the floor or table, and asked all three of us to try and move it with our minds. My dad told me later that I was the only one who moved the compass.

"Through my home schooling I learned about yoga and meditation, but also how to care for farm animals, and even how to shoot a gun. My dad was a Vietnam War veteran. Having him for a father taught me to be incredibly open-minded, as he was a bundle of contradictions. He'd had a checkered past, and suffered from Post-Traumatic Stress Disorder, yet he was completely dedicated to his children.

"My father died when I was twelve. Before he passed, our family life was similar in some ways to the 1970s TV sitcom *All in the Family*. When I was fifteen I participated in an internship program at Ananda Village for teens and young adults. I remember taking part in a lot of physical labor, falling in love for the first time, and feeling very included. We were all sitting out on the Village Green one evening, looking up at the stars and singing "Hallelu-jah" to the tune of Pachebel's Cannon. That was the first time I felt the joy in spirituality. I could feel myself breaking out of my shell.

"In retrospect, I couldn't have had a better upbringing. For many years I had tried to stuff myself into a box called 'normal.' It was only a matter of time before that box imploded. I was blessed, during my rebellious years, to be surrounded by supportive peers and adults.

"Now, my own eleven-year-old son is very psychic, and he's decided to be an atheist. You have to let your children walk their own path. They need to believe and explore whatever they need to explore. Sometimes children raised in a spiritual way can feel judged or inexperienced, so it's good for them to venture out into the world and walk and play.

"I didn't do well in school. After the terrorism of 9/11, I felt I needed to write poetry. I had an English teacher who understood me. She let me write poetry. She never singled me out, but when the opportunity presented itself, she knew how to draw me out.

"We need to learn not to impose our energy on our children, but help them navigate their own path. It's important to keep our needs and egos out of the way so that our children can blossom and discover who they are.

"Now, my livelihood is being a medium. I do readings for people. I have a message for them. I call myself a spiritual medium.

"Because we are identified with our physical bodies, it can be hard at first to connect with spiritual forms, such as meditation, prayer, and rituals. While working with people I tell them, whatever they experience, take what resonates deeply and use it.

"I remember going through a very challenging time in my life. My whole world was falling apart; nothing was working. Everything I did led to a dead end. After a few years of this I was worn down. Then something happened that was too much for me to handle. I had no money, no job, and didn't know where to turn. I sat down in my room and cried for a long time. After a long period of this I suddenly felt as if I were being pulled through the air. With lightning-like speed I was being drawn to a place in the Himalayas, and a voice spoke to me, saying, 'Ingrid, what is the matter? Don't you know I have always been with you?' There, in front of me, talking to me and consoling me, was the great avatar Babaji.*

---

* This great saint is described in *Autobiography of a Yogi*.

CHAPTER 8

When the Buddha Plays

"I believe all suffering is caused by ignorance. People inflict pain on others in the selfish pursuit of their happiness or satisfaction. Yet true happiness comes from a sense of brotherhood and sisterhood."
—His Holiness the 14th Dalai Lama,
12/10/89 Nobel Peace Prize Speech, Oslo, Norway

IN THE LATE NINETIES, a group of creative-minded adults involved with our community designed a performing arts summer camp. We planned to invite students between the ages of ten and seventeen to come together for a four-week intensive that would culminate with a dramatic production. Around this time, I had been reading the autobiography of the Dalai Lama, *Freedom in Exile*. His Holiness always referred to himself as "no one special," and "just a simple monk from Tibet." That book resonated deeply with many of us living in our yoga community.

In 1989 His Holiness was awarded the Nobel Peace Prize. In his acceptance speech, he said, "I believe the prize is a recognition of the true value of altruism, love, compassion and nonviolence which I try to practice, in accordance with the teachings of the Buddha and the great sages of India and Tibet." His Holiness was inspired by Mahatma Gandhi, who himself had led a nonviolent independence movement against British-ruled India from 1922 until his untimely assassination in 1948.

The plight of the Tibetans, and their desire to preserve their culture, seemed an ideal foundation for creating a stimulating educational and dramatic experience. During the nineties, plays about the Dalai Lama were not in vogue. But once this seed thought for the summer production was set, ideas began to unfold.

To deepen the students' understanding of Tibetan culture we decided to share with them the art of Tibetan masks used in ceremonial dances and operas performed in Himalayan monasteries. Creating a mask can be powerful and transforming for any person, so to understand this process I first created what I felt was a difficult mask to reproduce. It was the mask of a guardian Tibetan deity—black and red and quite fierce. It included a headdress of skulls, an eye in the middle of the forehead, and demonic teeth that were more like fangs. Ironically, these fierce masks are actually of benevolent Tibetan Gods who symbolize the courageous effort it takes to overcome evil. Sanskrit texts refer to these deities as *dharmapalas,* or "defenders of dharma."

The concept of warding off evil entered my life when our son was about four. I was intrigued by Jungian psychology and decided to introduce our boy to a Jungian sand tray therapist. Sand tray therapy is hands-on psychological work, and very healing. Using miniature statues selected from a vast menagerie displayed on shelves in the therapist's office, the child creates the sand tray while the therapist watches in silence. Through this mostly nonverbal experience, the therapist helps children actualize feelings they may not be able to express at a young age. The archetypal symbols serve as a bridge from the subconscious to the conscious, somewhat along the lines of bringing dreams into play.

As a way to help our son deal with the emotional aftereffects of open-heart surgery incurred when he was one year old, I scheduled an appointment. After leaving our son with the sand tray therapist for about forty-five minutes, I returned to her office to see what he had created. She took me into another room and proudly showed me his sand tray. My first reaction was, *Oh my gosh, what horrible creatures!* He had selected the most hideous monsters and dragons I'd ever seen. Some were on their feet in fighting stances with red eyes, bared teeth, and drooling tongues. He had arranged them all in a large circle. On the sides and in the middle were a few other objects. I looked at the therapist. "What does this mean?" She smiled softly and replied, describing the tray. "Oh it's very beautiful. You see, this is him in the center of the circle." I looked at the tiny object resting there. "He has surrounded himself with all these creatures because these are his guards, and they are there to protect him."

Though we must have talked on for several minutes, my mind coalesced around concepts that we use when sharing yoga philosophy with children. Though yogic adherents like Gandhi espoused nonviolence, courage, power, and strength are qualities that each soul can and must learn to express. The Bhagavad Gita and the Mahabharata are classical yogic epics that relate a multitude of battles and deaths, yet they serve as allegories for the age-old struggle between good and evil that takes place within our souls.

The Jungian concept of sand tray therapy would translate well into art projects. Working with the soft sculpting material needed to produce our Tibetan masks, I began to create some sample masks. I realized that, during the hot summer days, working with cool water and sculpting mud would become a visceral experience for the students. I would fill the art studio with images of Tibetan gods and goddesses, hang masks on the walls, and transform the room into a set from the ancient city of Lhasa. Buddhist chants and soft music would play in the background. And, just as the Sand Tray Therapist kept silence, I felt it was my duty to offer minimal instruction, to speak less and let each student find their inner Tibetan mask.

Before making the masks, we discussed the principles of courage, fending off evil, and protecting others. Some students felt drawn to being warriors, while others expressed themselves through masks that depicted animals or other deities.

The goddess of the Tibetan city of Lhasa is Sri Devi, the feminine wrathful deity, and the god of death is Yama, who holds the Tibetan wheel of life. There were many deities we could discuss. Tigers, monkeys, yaks, ibex, musk deer, and antelope would become part of the play as the wild animals of Tibet. Many Tibetan monasteries view the elusive snow leopard as a sacred animal, considering it a sin to kill these majestic creatures. Could the snow leopard have a role? Just as the Tibetan culture is slowly being lost, the vulnerable snow leopard remains an endangered species and a potent symbol.

Though modern plays and musicals have their own merit as entertainment, we were looking to accomplish more than the status quo. We wanted to create a deeply spiritual experience that would involve the students, the staff, and the audience. So we looked to world events that represented new shifts in consciousness. The awareness of many children born since the late eighties is more advanced than we realize. As teachers, we can intuit it. And thus, it helps children when higher qualities are modeled for them, and when they are surrounded by likeminded peers, teachers, and adults with higher awareness.

Our drama staff learned about His Holiness the Dalai Lama, his Tibetan history and spirituality, and we studied Tibetan Buddhist music, dance, and art. Then we came together and discussed our performing arts camp. What could we create that students of this age would relate to? What would be fun and memorable? We focused on the life of Buddha, drawing from Buddhist texts, but incorporating aspects of Tibetan Buddhism in art, mask-making, and dramatic dances.

The more we met together as a creative staff, the more the ideas matured. Each meeting began with a prayer and meditation. These group meditations helped keep us in tune with each other and our creative energies engaged. We ended by offering a prayer of unification for all those involved and the students we would serve.

As our ideas evolved, so did the cast of students who were meant to be part of this production. A group from Taiwan—a nation that decades ago achieved independence from Mainland China—would join our camp. This particular group had been exposed to yogic principles through ideals set forth by Joseph Cornell's Sharing Nature Foundation. The Taiwanese were well aware of the Dalai Lama, and many sympathized with the Tibetans' struggle for independence from Communist China. Students from the United States and Europe signed up. The camp would encompass learning about the Dalai Lama and Buddhism, and provide a time for deep cultural exchange. For those unfamiliar with Tibet's struggle for freedom, suffice it to say that even today, Mainland China continues to place pressure on those favoring His Holiness.

From our own yoga community and Living Wisdom School staff we drew qualified instructors in drama, music, art, and dance. We would have four weeks together—a short amount of time to produce a full-length play, with some students who could barely speak English. There would be dance rehearsals, drama auditions, music lessons, and art activities. And, each morning and evening, students and staff would engage in yoga, chanting, and meditation. Young college-aged students who had themselves attended a Living Wisdom School or Performing Arts Camp served with us to create a peer magnetism that was authentic. Several of these young interns also danced, acted, and sang in the play, building enthusiasm that spread quickly to the younger students.

A few of the dances we chose for this play, titled *The Life of Buddha*, included boys performing a Tai Chi-inspired warrior dance, girls twirling large colorful fans in a Chinese Fan Dance, and a Tibetan Cham Dance the students choreographed together. Traditionally, the Cham Dance was performed in medieval Tibetan Buddhist monasteries as a means of transforming the evils of the world into love and compassion. The costumes for that dance included the Tibetan masks the students had made in art classes. There were masks depicting Tibetan animals, nature spirits, and fierce gods and goddesses. One student constructed a mask four feet long and two feet wide. Some students danced, while others comprised an orchestra with violins, drums, and other instruments.

With only thirty days to pull together a quality production, the participants were under pressure. Those of us who had been busily choreographing, writing, directing, and helping to supervise, were challenged to the point of exhaustion. The twice-daily yoga and meditation sessions were oases of calm, and a welcome antidote for all the drama. Along the way were cultural exchanges of music, dance and cuisine; while group viewings of movies like *Little Buddha* and *Seven Years in Tibet* provided creative inspiration.

After nearly four weeks of preparation, the evening for the grand performance arrived. Our set for the play was an outdoor amphitheater surrounded by pine forests encircling Lotus Lake. A large stage, festive with hand-painted sets and colorful material, was situated in front of the lake. Above it all floated the conversations of young people, rising spontaneously from friendships growing closer.

It was just past dusk and the nearby forest grew darker. The time had come for the grand finale of *The Life of Buddha*. Crickets were humming. The sounds of bullfrogs chortling in the lake were reminiscent of Tibetan longhorns, sounding in the monasteries of India and Tibet.

The audience, seated in the sloping amphitheater facing the stage, hushed. From the left and right sides of the surrounding forest, lines of costumed Taiwanese, European, and American children appeared. They held candles and marched slowly, weaving towards the stage. The emerging darkness gave the lighted processional an ethereal glow. Their song was the six-syllabled mantra "Om Mani Padme Hum." Tibetan Buddhists believe that uttering this prayer invokes deep compassion. The words are engraved on the spinning prayer wheels the Tibetans hold sacred. It is said that the entire teachings of the Buddha are contained in the words Om Mani Padme Hum, their meaning beyond translation.

The Taiwanese have a very refined culture that values patience, humility, and friendship. The music their young students shared with us bore a level of sophistication beyond the performers' years. Though they spoke to us in broken English, the Taiwanese students showed the greatest courage in their efforts to communicate. I learned from them that placing the right hand over the left fist and raising both hands to your heart is a gesture of respect for the elders. Similarly, at Ananda, many of us greet each other with both hands folded as if in prayer: the yogic "namaste" of bowing to the highest in each other.

After the play, I approached the leader of the Taiwanese group, a teacher herself. I knew they would be leaving soon, right when our friendships were just beginning. How do you thank someone brave enough to bring a large group of youth from a small country like Taiwan to a yoga community in the forests of Northern California? I knew she felt as I did: we had done it all for the benefit of the students.

CHAPTER 9

When the Buddha Speaks

*"For the things we have to learn before we can do them,
we learn by doing them."* —Aristotle

IN MOST COLLEGES, ETHICS and values are not on the menu for required curriculum. In addition to the intellectual stimulation necessary to engage and train students, our yoga college honors an underlying theme of attunement and magnetism. In the fall of 2004 our college travel abroad group was searching for an adventure in Northern India. We were looking for some particularly magnetic events and people that had attunement to higher consciousness. We had been studying the Dalai Lama and his life for a course on World Cultures and Consciousness, when I reached out to His Holiness' office in India.

I was not expecting a response, but had the feeling a meeting with him would be a life-changing experience for our students. Six months later, through miraculous circumstances, I received an invitation for our college to have a private audience with His Holiness at his home in Mcleod Ganj, India, in March 2005. Our plans were to visit a number of holy people and sites to fulfill a study of world religions.

It's been said that students learn best in an experiential environment, and research proves this. We knew our yoga college needed to explore the world. What could we create that would speak to the highest ideals in young adults?

Values like courage, honesty, compassion, love, inner peace, service to others, and a sense of community were just a few of the qualities we focused on. To find and spend time with saintly people could be transformative for college students. Northern India is also the home of Mother Teresa of Calcutta, a venue many of our students longed to visit. Though she had had died eight years prior to our travel, our students were enthused about doing service projects at her missions of charity and her orphanage.

Calcutta is also the home of Yogananda, and many of his spiritual experiences chronicled in *Autobiography of a Yogi* took place there. It is also the home of Anandamoyi Ma, Ramakrishna and Vivekenanda, the poet Rabindranath Tagore, Aurobindo, and many other great souls. Then, too, we planned to visit a Sikh community near Delhi in order to understand Indian spiritual communities and the Sikh religion more thoroughly.

To discern the differences between Hinduism and Islam, we would meet with mystics, sadhus (ascetics), and swamis. Through our visit we hoped to become intimate with the major religions of Buddhism, Hinduism, Islam, Sikhism, and Catholic Christianity as they are practiced in India, a land where many great religions coexist harmoniously.

During one tour we became the first American college ever to meet with the religious studies department of the Islamic University in Delhi. It was only five years after the whole September 11 attack, and the negative propaganda that had been instigated made our students apprehensive about our visit. Before our departure we held many discussions about Islam and that terrorist event.

We contacted a Muslim professor from that university who was an interfaith adherent, and he helped set up meetings for us, a chance to worship together (the men and women separately), and to learn about their religion. Our first encounter was held in a faculty meeting room with the professors: all men plus one woman, staring at us. We were a bit awkward, and as I inwardly prayed for inspiration and guidance, I remembered something my teacher had said many years ago. "Try to find something in common with those you disagree with, or whose beliefs are very different from yours." So, knowing that the professors comprised a religious studies department, I asked if we could start the meeting with a prayer to the saints of all religions.

When I introduced ourselves to this faculty—our college, and our mission to learn more about other cultures—I stated that even though we had different ways of approaching God, at heart we all loved God, however-er strange our different belief systems may seem. That elicited warm smiles from all the Islamic professors. Our students asked questions—and we soon noticed the room filling up with Muslim students, many of them in full black burkas—they were curious about us. At one point, Nakula was looking at his cell phone when he noticed that a Muslim girl sitting next to him was looking at her phone too—we all laughed about it and the energy in the room relaxed even more.

Before our trip to see the Dalai Lama, our students had already toured Calcutta and Serampore, visited Sikh communities near Delhi, paid our re-spects to the Gandhi Memorial in Delhi, visited ashrams and Hindu shrines, and, before heading north to Rishikesh on the last part of our trip, visited with my teacher, Swami Kriyananda, at his home and ashram near Delhi. After Yogananda's passing in 1952, my teacher spent many years serving in India as a monk with his guru's organization, Self Realization Fellowship. He told me he had met with the Dalai Lama in 1959 in Delhi, shortly after His Holiness came from Lhasa to seek asylum in India. As my teacher was unable to travel with us to McLeod Ganj, he asked us to give His Holiness his love.

By the time we met with my teacher in February 2005, the cultural differences between India and America were triggering a variety of feelings among our students. One student asked how best to experience India. My teacher responded, "With your eyes closed and your hearts open."

In Rishikesh we met with Vanamali Devi, the Indian mystic and author who resided in a small ashram overlooking the Ganges River. From Rishikesh we planned our journey to "Little Lhasa," the Dalai Lama's home in McLeod Ganj, located in the far northwestern state of India, called Himachal Pradesh. All during our journey we'd been waiting to receive an email from His Ho-liness' secretary to let us know on which day and at what time our audience with him would occur.

As we looked at maps and discussed timeframes, the easier route would have been to take the train from Dehra Dun to Pathankot, and then taxi up to Dharamshala. We'd already spent a fair amount of time on the Indian railway, so we opted for a jeep trek from Rishikesh directly to McLeod Ganj. Students and faculty from the college would rendezvous in McLeod Ganj with students from the Living Wisdom High School, who were also traveling in India.

Our trip through the Himalayan foothills to see the Dalai Lama would take us through Simla, where we would overnight in an old hotel that hung to the cliffs and offered expansive views of the green mountains and forests that pushed towards the snowy peaks.

We spent long days and nights zigzagging through cliffs and foothills. We were at the mercy of our drivers, all of whom were totally composed. They sped through small towns and encampments, gunning and racing to keep up with our jeep caravan. At times the jeeps tossed us about like rag dolls. We catapulted westward through the potholes and dirt roads of Northern India. Indian buses and trucks, decorated like festive parades, sped by us. Around curves with thousand-foot mountain drops, we whirled.

Teashops and cafes were sparse, but our drivers instinctively sought them out. Just as we were approaching what seemed the hundredth mountain cliff, a herd of sheep and goats meandered slowly onto the road in front of us. Their owner tried to herd them quickly across, but to no avail. They baaed and bleated as we, captive in our metal machines, could feel their discontent. I turned to one of the students whose mouth was open. When driving on dirt roads in India, time is measured by patience, the number of potholes missed, and the sheer strength of one's lower back. We arrived at the old hotel in Simla late in the evening. After a brief meditation and a midnight snack, we retired to our rooms, melting into horizontal yoga postures with welcoming ease.

The next morning Nakula, checking the clock, herded us out the door after a bleak breakfast of tea and poori breads. He knew our "sheep" were getting anxious. After two twelve-hour days of mountain travel, we began to climb the road to Dharamshala, the home of the Dalai Lama. The population suddenly turned Tibetan. Deep burgundy robes trimmed in gold, worn by Tibetan Buddhist monks and nuns, appeared everywhere. Shaved heads reflected their certainty as they walked together in small groups. Like their eyes, their walk was direct and purposeful, their arms and calves muscular.

McLeod Ganj sits at the top of a crest of mountains, just beneath a few higher mountains, and with a view of the sylvan Kangra Valley below and the snow-capped Himalayas above. After a three-day journey (which seemed to take a month), our drivers began to surrender their pace. We drove slowly into town. The signs were now in Tibetan, and the majority of the population was Tibetan, though English and Sanskrit appeared throughout the mélange. Our jeeps stopped near the center of town, and we unpacked backpacks and suitcases. The drivers graciously helped us, then fled to the nearest teahouse.

The Pema Thang Guest House was a fifteen-minute walk from our drop-off. We passed stores full of Tibetan wares, hand-held prayer wheels, large-beaded Tibetan malas, and intriguing Thangka paintings that called to us.

On the surface, Little Lhasa was overpopulated, overflowing with the quiet dignity of a culture that had experienced massive suppression. The scene around us grew richer, as our tiny suitcase wheels knocked clumsily. Thick amber, silver, red, and turquoise beads adorned little stalls. Beneath us the old pavement was carved with random holes.

Ahead of us life-size Tibetan prayer wheels lulled followers in an open temple courtyard. The large wheels, called *mani*, were imprinted with numerous copies of the Om Mane Padme Hum mantra. We watched as old Tibetans strolled by them, running their fingers across the large wheels, twirling their cosmic prayers and mantras. They walked slowly, circumambulating so as to follow the direction of the sun. Tibetan Buddhists consider this ritual a spiritual practice. Metaphorically, one is turning the wheels of dharma (right action) and invoking blessings from an enlightened being who is the embodiment of compassion.

The rooms of the Pema Thang Guest House were simple, a few single beds with heavy woolen blankets, small bathrooms with showers and buckets. Each room looked out onto a steep hillside with trees and buildings colliding above a large yellow temple. Tibetan prayer flags were everywhere. Though it was March and still quite cold, we opened the windows. The deep drones of Tibetan monks chanting in the temple below drifted up. Their sounds were low, guttural, coming from the throat—long notes of OM linked continuously. Occasionally, the notes would vary an octave higher. At times it seemed like the growl of wild animals, an unearthly yet mystical chorus. Bells, drums, and Tibetan longhorns occasionally played.

A Tibetan lama had initiated this form of chanting over five hundred years ago in a monastery in Lhasa, Tibet. It has been preserved here, where the Dalai Lama of Tibet now lives in exile, a foundation for spiritual awakening. We held our own group meditation and chanting, and contemplated our environment. In the evening we headed to the Pema Thang Café, located in the front of the guest house. We ordered traditional Tibetan momo: steamed dumplings floating in a hearty vegetarian soup.

In the days leading up to our visit with His Holiness, we visited with a few scholars and Tibetan activists, interviewing and engaging them. The Free Tibet movement resonated deeply with our students. Free Tibet signs and tee shirts were everywhere, and our students were intrigued. We did our best to connect them with everything Tibetan. We visited orphans at the Tibetan Children's Village, spent time in their schools, and listened to refugees who had escaped from Tibet to McLeod Ganj. In many ways this town was a spiritual community reestablishing itself in a new world. The weariness in the eyes of many of the elders held a calmness born of sacrifice.

On the morning we were to see His Holiness, we rose early, did some energizing exercises, then meditated. Before rising we could hear the deep chanting of the monks, floating up from the Dalai Lama's temple, a soothing wake-up bell for our own practices.

The Dalai Lama keeps a strict discipline. He rises early and, before 5:00 a.m., has finished his prostrations, chanting, and meditation. Tibetan Buddhist prostrations are vigorous and typically completed many times. One starts from a standing position, then kneels, then stretches full-length on the floor. The arms are fully extended above the head, with palms resting flat with fingers extended up towards the ceiling. Then, bending the knees and returning to the standing position, one places one's palms pressed together on the crown of the head, then brings them down to the heart.

After breakfast we headed down towards the temple. On the way, we stopped at the Tibetan Museum. With anticipation of our meeting, we did our best to keep in silence. We walked slowly through the museum, located above the Dalai Lama's main temple.

Our walking meditation brought us past hundreds of displays, photos, and brief videos chronicling the Tibetan uprising, the invasion by China, and His Holiness' last trip by horse and mule along the ledges of the Tibetan Himalayas during his escape to India. Tibet had been a small, religious, and independent nation, led, starting in 1951, by a young Dalai Lama. Though there had been prior acts of aggression against the Tibetans, in 1950 the newly established Communist regime proclaimed that Tibet must become part of the People's Republic of China. Shortly after, they invaded the small nation.

From 1950 to 1951, the Chinese People's Liberation Army continued their invasion, which was characterized by acts of murder, torture, and rape, and cruel and inhumane treatment. It is estimated that more than a million Tibetans were murdered during the Chinese occupation. In one year alone, from 1959–60, eighty-seven thousand lives were lost. Monks and nuns were imprisoned by the Chinese for their religious views and their loyalty to the Dalai Lama. Even today, nuns are raped in Chinese prisons and images of the Dalai Lama are banned. There was no chance of keeping the Tibetan culture alive with the Chinese in control. Monasteries had been burned, scholars tortured, and atrocities committed in the name of power.

(Today, in 2017, I visited with a young Chinese physics student studying yoga at our community. I asked her whether China's communist regime had lessened. She shook her head and said that China's leadership still disavows religion, or anything considered spiritual.)

The Tibetan Museum serves as an important vehicle that captures truth. It is the largest Tibetan research archive in the world, a document for past and future generations. Since the invasion, ethnic Chinese have been encouraged to occupy Tibet. The Chinese have elected their own heir to Tibetan Buddhism, in an effort to further suppress the Dalai Lama's followers.

Little Lhasa captivated us. Orphanages, schools, businesses, and monasteries exist here in stark contrast to another world far away in the high plateaus of the Himalayas. The trip to the museum was sobering, providing more questions than answers. Our sense of outrage was stifled by the imminence of our next appointment. The Dalai Lama's temple called to us from the slopes below.

He is considered to be the reincarnation of each of the previous thirteen Dalai Lamas of Tibet—all said to be manifestations of Avalokiteshvara: The Bodhisattva of Compassion and Bearer of the White Lotus. The white lotus is a symbol of purity in Vedic culture, from whence both Hinduism and Buddhism have evolved. Both paths have their roots in the subcontinent of India, though new branches have emerged, grown, and modified over many thousands of years. It is fitting that India, home to Hinduism or Sanaatan Dharma, the oldest religion in the world dating back four thousand years, opened its arms to the Dalai Lama when he fled his country in 1959.

At the Dalai Lama's residence, we went through intense security before we were shown to His Holiness' living room. Finally, we all filed in. Included in our group were a few other college-age Westerners studying Buddhism. His Holiness jumped up from his seat and walked over to us with the warmth of a young child meeting a long-lost friend. His aura was magnetic, large, and completely captivating. He smiled and chortled, greeting us and allowing us to interact with him up close. The Dalai Lama was very childlike, with no pretenses—all smiles and intense inner joy.

He was instantly drawn to one of our students: a tall Chinese-American teen, of the Hare Krishna following, with a shaved head and single pony tail. An array of religious beads were draped around the student's wrists and neck. The Dalai Lama smiled broadly at him. He examined the student's clothing and gestured to his tiny ponytail, asking "What's this?" He then chuckled while surveying every detail of the young man's clothing, as if admiring an exotic animal. His Holiness spoke little English; nonetheless, he continued to engage the young student.

Beneath his burgundy robes, trimmed in gold, the Dalai Lama's arms were quite muscular. His physique was strong and strident, its fierceness softened by a face that appeared both fatherly and motherly. He beheld us all. His eyes and smile are in perfect attunement, permanently etched, changing momentarily while speaking of serious matters. Even then, he brought levity and humility to our most serious questions. He was completely down-to-earth and unaffected.

We had ten questions for the Dalai Lama, which we had sent to him before our visit. As we prodded him with our inquiries, it was clear than in spite of all the outward misfortune of the invasion of his country, the suppression of Tibetan Buddhism, and the continuous onslaught against him, His Holiness held no animosity towards the Chinese. He was an untethered sprite who had escaped the very thing the Chinese seem bent on condemning him for—his spiritual leadership of the Tibetan Buddhist people. He laughed as he acknowledged that the Chinese would prefer his death, saying, "Chinese cannot kill Dalai Lama." Then he laughed even harder, his head ducking and bowing. Of course, we understood that he was referring to the reincarnation teaching that the soul never really dies.

I had heard that the Dalai Lama pays close attention to Westerners. I remembered reading, too, that he loves watches. During our visit I observed that he was wearing a large gold watch. I was sitting right next to him. Normally I don't wear a watch, but on that day I sported a small inexpensive Timex. I noticed him looking at my wrists. On my right wrist I wore an astrological bangle made of three metals, the same type that Sri Yukteswar had prescribed for Yogananda. I was reminded of Yukteswar's words to Yogananda; "By a number of means—by prayer, by will power, by yoga meditation, by consultation with saints, by use of astrological bangles—the adverse effects of past wrongs can be minimized or nullified."*

We asked the Dalai Lama to recall a memorable time in his life. He harkened back to the occasion when he and his younger brother Tenzin Choegyal visited Mao Tse-Tung in 1954 in Beijing. Tenzin was good at mimicking people. During their visit Mao stepped out for a bit, and Tenzin began imitating him, much to the Dalai Lama's amusement. His brother was still doing this

---

* Paramhansa Yogananda, *Autobiography of a Yogi* (Nevada City, California: Crystal Clarity Publishers, 2005), 164.

when Mao returned to the room, standing right behind him so he couldn't be seen. His Holiness was laughing as he told us this story, sometimes bent over in his chair, he was laughing so hard. He was in tears. We all laughed with him. It was hard not to. The Dalai Lama had brought us into his heart and helped us feel his mirth, his happiness, his childlike joy.

He continued with the story. Instantly the two Tibetan brothers thought they were in trouble, having offended Chairman Mao. Then Mao laughed because he too thought that Tenzin's imitation of him was funny—so they all began laughing. The brothers were relieved that they weren't going to get decapitated or ousted for this behavior.

When I reflect on our time together, His Holiness was trying to relax all of us, his college visitors. Later I read that he said Chairman Mao was one of the most influential people he'd ever met, because Mao offered him some very useful advice on how to lead people.

The world's most famous monk was graciously spending time with all of us. We had one final question. "What advice would you give to a small spiritual college like ours?" "Keep doing what you're doing. Travel the world and experience other religions and cultures. Go out and see how they live." Through these simple words, and with his enormous love, the Dalai Lama christened our inaugural voyage abroad for the college.

Our time was coming to a close. His attendants invited us into the court-yard, where he humbly presented us with white Tibetan scarves that he blessed. Bowing to each one of us, and we to him, he draped a scarf around each neck. Afterwards we gathered for a photograph with him in the yard of his home.

It's been over twelve years since our meeting with His Holiness. The white scarf he'd given me still surrounds a large photo of Yogananda in our medita-tion room. In our college Library of Higher Consciousness, a cheerful color portrait of His Holiness smiles at passersby, a simple reminder of the soul's need to look beyond the horrors of this earth plane and practice forgiveness, the ultimate expression of compassion for all.

It has been said that great saints exude a childlike innocence. As we at-tuned to His Holiness that day, we all wanted to laugh and play. He has that effect on people, a spontaneous reaction to the purity and innocence of his heart. He's been called the Holder of the White Lotus, the Ocean of Wisdom, Protector of the Land of Snows, the Mighty of Speech, a Living Buddha, and Tibet's Wish-Fulfilling Gem. Though he says he might not reincarnate again, it is written that The Bodhisattva of Compassion will return to earth for eternity to help ease the suffering of humankind.

It was time to leave. We hauled our tiny suitcases back to the center of town. As we neared the large prayer wheels, we set suitcases aside, approached the wheels, and spun our final prayers, circumambulating along with the Tibetans. At the center of town, we loaded our gear onto an all-night bus headed for Delhi. Once again we were jerked and thrown as we raced down the steep curves from McLeod Ganj. I caught the eye of one of the students as a particularly sharp curve hurtled us several feet off our seats. Eight hours later we landed in Delhi. We spent time at the Ananda Sangha ashram for a day. Then, in the middle of the night, our taxis were racing once again, this time to Indira Gandhi International Airport. We were on our way home.

"For as long as space endures, and for as long as living beings remain, until then may I, too, abide to dispel the misery of the world."

—A traditional Buddhist prayer, quoted by His Holiness the Dalai Lama in his autobiography, *Freedom in Exile*

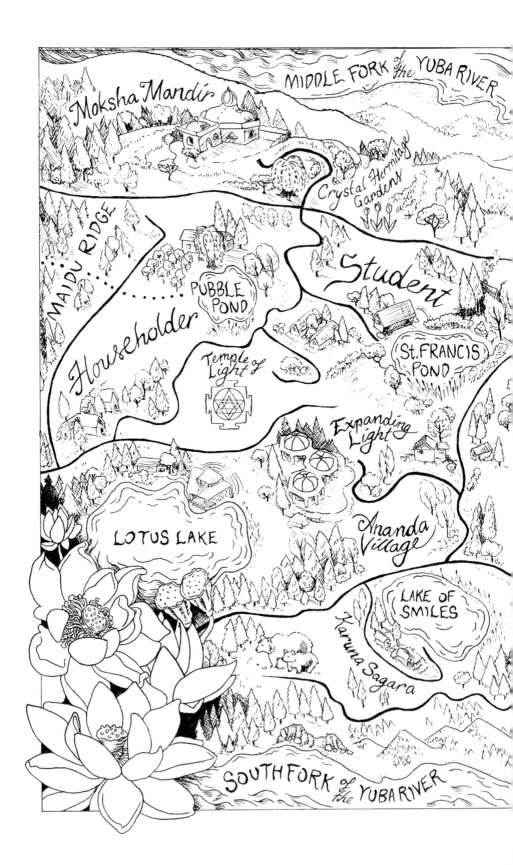

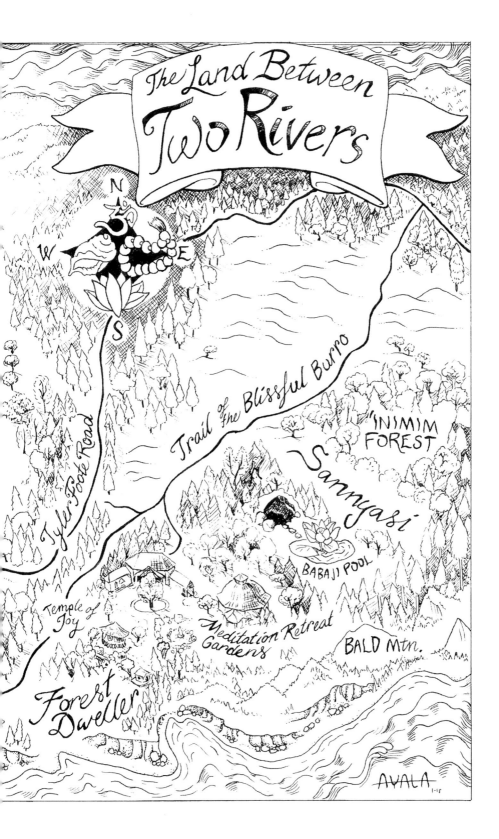

CHAPTER 10

The Householder—Age 24–48

In this fictionalized story, lotus flowers and a cottage inhabited by the Hindu goddess Lakshmi offer esoteric wisdom for the second stage of yoga.

A PLEASANT WIND BLOWS IN from the south. The milky sky of summer is lighting on the red roof of a small cottage. The simple home with green shutters and a white portico overlooks a landscape of lush gardens interwoven by trails that lead to other cottages. A nearby small community encircles a blue-domed temple crowned with golden lotus-shaped flowers.

To the north is a winding river, running wild. To the south is another river. Between the two rivers is a householder community.

In front of the house, a yogini is seated on the portico in lotus posture. In symbolic tribute to the divine nature of Lakshmi, the yogini has two sets of arms, indicative of her celestial ability to outwit the cosmic forces of delusion. Her upper right hand is held up, palm facing outward, blessing all who enter. In her upper left hand she holds a mala given to her during the student stage, awarded to her as a symbol of her daily meditation discipline. In her lower right hand she holds a long-stemmed red lotus flower, symbol of her steadfast devotion to the Divine. In her lower left hand she holds a white lotus, given to her by her beloved as a reminder of her purity and her vows.

Lakshmi's offering of the lotus flowers symbolizes the inner offering by each devotee of renewal, fertile creativity, and supreme divinity, sprouting from the mud of the earth plane to bloom and soar in eternal bliss. The lotus is the symbol for the householder stage of life. As we enter this stage we recognize that we have grown beyond the rigors of youthful discipline, that have kept us physically strong, and are now preparing to blossom—each of us according to our unique karma. The green leaves of the lotus wave like great fans upon the water, spreading ripples in all directions—a symbol of our own adventurous energy. Lotus buds stand tall and attentive like young householders.

The unfolding lotus tells a story of rich, exciting, outward flowing energy. The householder stage is associated with the southern direction, the color red, the season of summer, mature youth, and the outward energy of growth. The psychoanalyst Carl Jung describes this stage as the time of the warrior, the time to set goals, to reinvent ourselves, and to conquer the world.

The householder stage is magnetically charged with warmth, strength, and physical beauty. Now is the time to find a mate, a successful career, a first apartment, then a home for children and family life, and a network of close friends who share our ideals. It is the time of weddings, families, and living in communities. The Indian mystic Vanamali Devi says that many people are hypnotized by the householder stage, and never leave. For yogi householders the task is to learn to serve others. We do so through our own family, until we learn to transcend the family unit and serve all, just as the sannyasi does.

The householder stage is also the time that work and career lead us into creative adventures. Through their careers, yogis can be models of strong work ethics and virtues, so much needed in today's businesses. Engagement with career and friends provides its own satisfaction.

If we remain single during this stage, what we do has the potential to help us grow towards greater understanding, maturity and inner happiness. If we have chosen to live as a monastic, we see all our actions as an offering to the Divine.

Just as within the lotus flower, so deep inside our heart resides a small golden light representing the immortal Atman. Our higher Self, God within, dwells within this light. Having learned the discipline of meditation during the first stage of yoga, we are now ready to experience the deeper lessons of the heart.

For householders as well as for monastics, the route home is the same.

Yogananda was once asked this question: "I understand you have two classes of students: those who live in the world, and those who live in the monastery as renunciates. Which of these two ways do you consider the better, and why?" Yogananda answered, "Good, better, and best are determined by the depth of one's love for God. Outside of divine devotion, nothing else matters."[*]

---

[*] Swami Kriyananda, *Conversations with Yogananda* (Nevada City, California: Crystal Clarity Publishers, 2004), 335.

CHAPTER 11

Gita's Way

THIRTEEN WEEKS PREGNANT AND expecting her second child, Gita is sitting at her desk where she leads nonprofit development for a large yoga organization. She is firmly in the Householder Stage of Yoga, the most active outward time. I asked her how yoga has influenced her life. "The teachings of yoga have helped me to see my role as a parent—bringing a little soul into the world—as a way of deepening my love, but also bringing me to a deeper sense of nonattachment. I'm beginning to understand there's something bigger happening, and understanding that allows me to be more centered. With my eighteen-month-old daughter, I'm constantly challenged to be more centered, to create boundaries, and I'm learning to say 'no.'"

One of the main things Gita is learning right now is how to share the same love she has for her family with God. "There was a time in my growing understanding of nonattachment when I realized I wasn't the center of my parent's world—God was—and I was angry about that." Gita has had the rare blessings of being born into a family where yoga philosophy is understood and practiced. Even her name, which means "song" in Sanskrit, is drawn from the famous Bhagavad Gita, the "Song of God." "As a child of two yogi parents, it took me a long time to realize what my parents were trying to do.

"For older children and young adults, growing up can bring feelings of not being wanted, feelings brought on by the wanting of the familial closeness most of us had as young children. I think every child has this experience, except for those with helicopter parents," she laughed.

I was curious if growing up in a yoga community, then leaving, was similar to the experience of Native Americans who left the reservation. Would they fall into darkness, their lives tainted by worldly American culture? If they returned to the reservation, how would they cope with problems of reintegration? How would they deal with shunning, or lack of support from their tribe?

What was it like to be born in a spiritual community, leave the community, then come back thirteen years later? Some children who grew up in a community left and never returned. Some came back. Some remained friendly or lived nearby. Some started their own small communities. Perhaps some disliked their experience. Perhaps others are somewhere far away, still trying to integrate their experience.

"So, what was it like to grow up in a yoga community? I asked Gita. "It was bliss," she answered. "Yes, it was heaven on earth. It was so safe and full of loving happy people that you could have freedom in a way other children in the world couldn't. At Ananda Village we had an eight-hundred-acre playground. We were outside in nature a lot. There were no strangers." Gita reminisced about her friendships with adults too. "There's a natural and genuine level of trust here and a certain innocence that doesn't exist in the outside world." I wondered what it would feel like for a young girl, to grow up in a bubble—isolated from the world beyond community. "Adults with different skills were brought into our schools and often mentored us as well. People were genuine. We called adults and teachers by their first names. There were no titles like 'Mister this' or 'Miss that.'"

I asked Gita how life at Ananda was different from living in a small town. "The difference is that the people who are here have chosen to be here and truly want to be here. The residents share similar values—for example, the community prohibition against alcohol and drugs. All the adults are meditating and striving to be better people." When she was thirteen, Gita moved to Seattle with her parents and attended her first public school. "I was a total country bumpkin," she said. "But I was genuinely myself, so my classmates took pity on me. I felt like I was living a scene out of *Napoleon Dynamite*. One day I was in the school lunchroom with hundreds of other students. I was walking with my tray; I tripped and the tray went flying." Fortunately, a girl scooped her up and helped her.

"I became good friends with the students in band and theatre because they seemed the most real. They were passionate about what they did and they weren't afraid to be geeks or to be genuinely themselves," she said. Public school had its own flaws. "I experienced racism for the first time." One of her close friends began wearing tee shirts touting Asian Pride. "I was offended by the fact that race had become a differentiator for friendship," she added.

Though her parents remained in Seattle, when she was sixteen she moved back to the yoga community and lived with two different families. Living in the community had its own drawbacks: "I had preacher's kid syndrome and soon began to rebel." At one time her rebellion almost got her kicked out of the community. Not living at home with her parents gave her leeway to rebel. "When I was a kid, I gobbled up meditation and chanting. I meditated in my parent's meditation room. I have memories of growing up that were akin to magic. But I had to rebel. From sixteen to nineteen I started smoking cigarettes, I became self-conscious and worried about my appearance. I began experimenting with alcohol and marijuana. I think I had to rebel to begin to figure out what I really cared about," she explained.

To begin to put her life in order, Gita first rejected everything, and then began the search for what really mattered. She attended Pepperdine in Malibu and got her BA in International Studies. Later she got her MA in Nonprofit Administration from the University of San Francisco. "The job market after graduation was difficult, but by the time I was twenty I was through with my rebellion," she said. "I worked as a nanny, traveled to Italy, and finally, turning back to yoga, studied Raja Yoga," she continued.

What she really wanted to do, though, was to use her life to help people. I asked Gita what it was that brought out her altruistic streak. During her childhood in the yoga community Gita had an experience that helped to shape her future: "Between the ages of five and twelve I worked with a woman who kept rescued horses and ponies." The woman lived nearby, and Gita was able to earn money by cleaning the horse stalls and helping to care for the horses. She eventually earned three hundred dollars, bought an abused pony, retrained her; in turn, the ponies helped train Gita: "There's something wonderfully heart-opening about working with horses. Having a relationship with such a highly intuitive animal changed me."

The daily experience with her horse helped Gita develop an intangible closeness with another being. Together with another girl who had her own rescue horse, Gita would take early morning rides through the hills of the community. Many young girls were part of a pony club the community had developed. "I had a particular relationship with Cassie, a very intuitive rescue horse," she remarked. "After riding her for a while I learned that all I had to do was barely lean one way or another and Cassie would turn." I asked her to elaborate, explain what it was like. "It's like surfing. There's something spiritual about it. You feel as though you're on a wave and you're one with the ocean. You're riding and doing something with another being—no words between you, but you get to share something deeply."

She continued. "As an adult, you seek unity with your partners, but as a kid you seek it in the world around you." Each horse, like each human, has a unique personality. "There was a Shetland Pony named Moonstone who had the habit of running very fast, then stopping dead in her tracks," she said. "I always felt that, in her own way, she was playing with me," she laughed.

During her college years, Gita's interest in International Studies began to ignite her desire to help suffering people in other countries. Many years after college graduation, she landed a job with CARE, the international organization that helps struggling nations.

"After forty-five years of existence, the CARE organization had established a very large reach." Besides offering a deep culture of learning what people really need and how they can be helped in a longer rhythm, CARE was also fulfilling Gita's humanitarian desires. One of her favorite projects at CARE was a Maternal Health Program established for indigenous women in the back country of Peru.

"The indigenous women were having high maternal fatality rates because, when they were ready to deliver their babies, if they had pregnancy complications, they often couldn't get to the hospital in time. Unfortunately, the hospitals weren't sensitive to the cultural birth practices of the indigenous women, whose traditional practice of squatting to give birth conflicted with hospital protocol of lying down to give birth," she explained.

"CARE created birthing centers closer to the indigenous villages so that needed supplies would be readily available. They trained the local midwives in sanitation and other practices," said Gita. Instead of having to take a full day to reach a hospital, a pregnant woman could reach a CARE birthing center in only two hours: "These care centers were located at midpoints between the villages and the hospitals, to shorten the journey should the woman need further care."

Her work with CARE gave Gita a way to give back to communities, especially significant because it was growing up in a yoga community that had first nurtured her native altruism: "My idealism came from my experiences with the Ananda Schools. We always had altruistic projects that I loved. In the early nineties, when environmental causes were of great concern, the school children raised money to adopt a wild humpback whale. We did all sorts of fun things to deepen our awareness of environmental issues. Besides helping scientists who protected endangered species, the children raised money to buy three acres of rainforest in South America."

One of Gita's life-shaping experiences came when a group of the school's students traveled to Mexico to help in an orphanage. The students all learned Spanish before they embarked on their trip. Once at the orphanage, they lived right alongside the young orphans and did everything they did. For two weeks they ate the same rice and beans the orphanage children ate at every meal. They cleaned and did chores together. They forged friendships and did projects together. Gita reflected, then said, "This experience really helped shape who I am."

<h1 style="text-align:center">Chapter 12</h1>

How Couples Become

My teacher once said the relationship of the ideal couple is like that of brother and sister. There may be romantic love and sexuality in the beginning; when all that is stripped away, what remains is friendship. Yogananda urged his students to seek out friends from past incarnations to perfect those friendships. "One lifetime is not always sufficient to achieve such perfection."[*]

∽

Yogananda offered a prayer for those earnestly seeking their life partner. For those wishing to attract a true soul partnership, Yogananda offered the following affirmation, to be practiced daily, after meditation: "Heavenly Father, bless me that I choose my life companion according to Thy law of perfect soul union." After meditation say it loudly a few times, then more softly, then whispering, then mentally, then subconsciously, and finally superconsciously. Work with this affirmation for at least six months, with deep faith. Through using this affirmation, and attunement to God, one will find a suitable companion. If you have been drawn towards an inharmonious companion, Yogananda said God will bring about circumstances that will prevent your making a wrong choice.

---

[*] Paramhansa Yogananda, *How to Love and Be Loved* (Nevada City, California: Crystal Clarity Publishers, 2007), 54.

One friend told me how she met her future husband. She had grown tired of failed relationships and wanted something that would work: "I told Yogananda that I needed his guidance; my way of doing this was to write him a letter." In the letter she listed all the qualities she wanted in a partner and asked Yogananda for his help. Two days later a new friendship began, though at the time it was not romantic. "We got along great and were having fun just being friends. I never expected anything else." After quite some time her friend asked her about getting closer. "You mean marriage?" she asked him. "Well, yes," he replied. "Are you proposing to me?" she said. "Well, yes," he answered. Today they have a wonderful marriage and friendship.

Another friend met her future husband while doing something they both liked very much—hiking. Through their common interest they planted seeds for a deeper relationship that has lasted many years. To one woman, after she'd been praying for guidance about marriage, a divine voice spoke: "You don't get married because your relationship is already perfect. You get married to learn how to love!"

For those needing guidance with their marriage, Yogananda offers a prayer affirmation. One woman found great comfort in this prayer when she and her husband were encountering difficulties in the early years of her marriage: "Divine Mother, keep me and my husband (wife) perfectly united on the physical, mental, and spiritual planes. And may we live in a state of ever-increasing happiness by following Thy perfect laws. Aum, Peace, Amen."

In India many couples have different gurus or beliefs, and yet their marriages remain solid.

For many years, since she was the age of twelve, Nakula and I have had a relationship with an "adopted" daughter who was raised Hindu in India. By adopted I do not mean that we have papers or legal custody. Our relationship began when she came to one of our Living Wisdom Performing Arts Camps, grew steadily deeper when she came later to Ananda College, and has continued to grow during ongoing visits.

When she returned to India, we wondered if she might meet someone and fall in love. A few years later she announced to us that her mother and father had selected a man for her to marry. The Westerner inside me panicked: "But aren't you going to get to know him first and see if you really do like each other?" Instead of answering my question directly, there was silence. She began to tell me about the whole selection process. Intrigued, I started to look forward to meeting this young man. As her surrogate parents, our main concern was for her happiness and well-being.

In traditional Hindu families, the woman's parents select the husband for the daughter based on knowledge of the potential groom's family and a range of qualities that go into making a successful marriage. One of the most important determining factors is to have an expert study the Vedic astrological charts for the prospective bride and groom. Vedic astrology is considered more "predictive" than Western astrology; in India especially, Vedic astrology is taken very seriously.

A Vedic astrologer has a list of ten main qualities that make up a successful marriage. Our young friend told us that astrological chart analysis had found for her a successful match.

In ancient India, marriage was understood from a higher perspective. When a young couple reached marriageable age, the families of potential partners would discuss the availability of the son or daughter for marriage. Because marriages are believed to be made in the heavens, the analysis of the horoscope of each potential couple has enormous potential. Next would come the casting of the Vedic horoscope for each potential partner based on each criteria:

a. Varna Koota: The nature of the individual, whether the person is soft or aggressive.

b. Vashna Koota: The mutual attraction between the couple.

c. Yoni Koota: The sexual compatibility of the couple.

d. Taara Koota: The health and well-being of the couple.

e. Graha Maitri: The spiritual and intellectual levels of the couple.

f. Gana Koota: The temperament of the couple.

g. Rashi Koota: The emotional compatibility of the couple.

h. Naadi Koota: Indicates the health internally and externally (pitta, kapha, vata: the three fundamental biological energies) in their bodies.

The astrological point system has a maximum of thirty-six; if a couple gets eighteen or more points the marriage is considered compatible. Southern Indian astrologers also look at the longevity of the marriage, potential children and grandchildren, the duration of married life, and the couple's ability to drive away misfortune.

In Vedic lore, the marriage ritual often signifies a couple beginning their second cycle of life—the householder stage. As an accompaniment to this ritual, the groom may take the bride out under the night sky to ask for the blessings of Vashistha and Arundhati—twin stars that rotate in synchronicity. The synchronized movement of these two stars signifies the ideal marriage. Just as both of these stars orbit the same center and travel through space together, so the yogic couple can help each other evolve their mutual love and devotion.

A Vedic astrologer friend completed what he called a "composite chart" for my husband and me before we were married. Our charts showed that we had been together many lifetimes. The advice he gave us for our marriage has proven to be quite accurate. When we met we both had independent natures. We each owned our own business and had employees. Because we were committed to our yogic path, and so were looking for ways to begin our life together in a conscious way, our Vedic astrologer's perspective gave us impersonal ways to harmonize our independent natures and work together on our shared journey. Later in our marriage, when our son came, Vedic astrology helped us understand his life directions as well.

CHAPTER 13

Family Yoga

Peak summer brought heavy fog to the coastal town of Cambria. It surrounded our home in a blanket so icy and penetrating that my father would rise early, usually at five, gather kindling, cautiously arranging each piece, and make an art of placing wood in the old stone fireplace that was the central heating.

As the fire began to rumble and spit, the golden blaze rolled higher and captured him; my father would sigh and lean back in his chair to tend it. An ornate poker hanging precariously from a large hook became his sword, guiding how to make flames last, which log to add, and when to let the coals timber down. My mother would bring her coffee to join him, pulling up a chair next to his. In silence they would watch the flames.

After their morning ritual, the nest warm, mother would begin the long process of making bread, lining the table with waxed papers and flour, timing the dough, waiting, rolling, folding, then anointing the soft baguettes that would gently bake in her oven. Outside, the chickens were begging for cornmeal; the garden, full in July, was beckoning. With the fog still clinging, she pursued the tiny paths of her French intensive garden, tracking insects and predators, pulling the weeds that challenged her greens, imagining how the children might help her work the acre of bounty. She examined artichokes, surveyed carrots, and nudged tomatoes, while recipes of pottages and soups aligned themselves in her mind. Walking to a long clothesline, she rearranged pieces needing the sun's attention. Then, scooting inside to greet the early risers, she and my father announced the day.

There were tasks to explain and lists to read; as the dining room filled, we sleepy children all knew to listen carefully. My father would set on the table a large bottle of milk fresh from a friend's cow; he would explain that he would be bartering, offering a gift in exchange, perhaps something my mother had made, or abalone from the ocean, or a large burlap bag of pinecones we'd collected nearby, ideal for fire.

He would open the milk container, carefully skim the thick cream off the top into a jar, our eyes following every move. "And we know what this is for," he would smile mischievously, and, reciting a humorous limerick, hand it to my mother. Hot buckwheat groats were served, fresh milk ladled on top, each meal beginning with a prayer led by a different family member. "Rub a dub dub, thanks for the grub. Yay, God!" the young family comedian would start; my mother would raise one eyebrow and, giving him a sidelong glance, smile, then laugh out loud.

It was Saturday and there was work to be done. Carrying bowls, one team would head to the nearby forest, combing the ground for wild strawberries and early mushrooms. Others would help mother weed and harvest the garden; an older brother, wanting to build his muscles, would dig trenches in the garden, clip hedges and bushes, and split logs and kindling for the fire. Some would scavenge for abalone in the nearby ocean: a full day of work wading or swimming in freezing tidal pools.

One child would assist with the laundry, adding soap and warm water to a small electric washer, then rinsing, before finally piling the wet clothes in a large basket. The final task, operating the hand wringer, was the favorite— watching as the rollers chewed each tee shirt, removing the precious water my mother would gather carefully for the garden.

We lived in an area of perpetual drought: Even the dew from clinging fog nourished the garden. When the sun arrived at noon, we'd quickly hang out the laundry, and haul it in before fog enfolded us again. We worked with nature. If our foraging produced enough tiny strawberries, my mother would make homemade strawberry shortcake with heavy whipping cream for an evening treat. After dinner there were dishes to be washed and rinsed by hand, floors to be swept, laundry to be brought in, and wood to be stacked for the fire.

The evening fire was prepared, with father coaching and tending, mother soaking pinto beans for the next day. Baths were gauged by water availability; then all gathered in the living room, five pairs of pajamas sprawled on the carpet, ready for the nightly story. As we watched the blazing fire, father read from Rudyard Kipling, or adventure tales and poetry about places that coaxed our dreams. Gradually, one by one, each child headed to bed, exhausted from the day's work, enlivened by the love and energy that encircled us.

Two of the gifts my parents gave were simple living and learning how to work together as a family. As Nakula and I patched together work, career, and family, there were new challenges.

After putting baby Rama down to bed, I'd sneak into the meditation room, ironically wedged between his room and ours. Sitting to meditate, I'd practice several minutes of pranayama breathing exercises, a toehold on inner peace. Then I would shift to my deeper practice of Kriya Yoga. That's when it would start. First, a few squawks from the nursery. The squawks would get louder, the long-winded cries all parents know will inevitably lead to screams emitted from something that's being tortured, or perhaps held over a steep cliff with no chance of survival. *Ah, well, I didn't really need that meditation after all.*

After nearly two years of countless meditation interruptions, my husband very sweetly suggested I might like to go into seclusion for a few days while he watched the baby. *This is your first baby, and it might be your only baby.* Before marriage it was easy to meditate for three hours and longer. Once married, to keep harmony in the household we had to adjust our schedules, to make sure we had at least one daily meditation together. When disharmony came or communication weakened, we knew why. Meditating together offers couples inner attunement and communication that goes beyond words.

During the householder phase, meditation routines are constantly rearranged. Perhaps it was this constant pressure on the couple's spiritual life that lay behind Yogananda's recommendation to have smaller families, even suggesting only one child. What helped us was our intention to meditate, our commitment to meditation as a priority. When we couldn't meditate because of life-threatening family distractions (they all *seemed* life-threatening), we did something simpler, like singing together or cooking a breakfast together, sharing love in a meaningful way. If our family was struggling and the morning I wanted to have a long meditation it wasn't possible, intuition became my guide. If my intention was true, another meditation time would surface.

Worrying about missed meditation or family problems creates more stress. Allowing children to join meditations is wonderful, when they choose to, and can be very comforting. Seeing their parents meditate together every day sends positive messages to children. Over time they feel the peace themselves, and someday may use meditation to their own benefit. Forcing them to meditate or giving material rewards for good behavior can backfire. Love and kindness are the best rewards: They are expressions of what your children want most—your affection and your energy.

One young woman I interviewed enjoyed meditating when she was a child. She'd join her mother when she was meditating, sitting next to her or even in her lap, the energy soothing and calming her. Today she is an accomplished yoga teacher. Perhaps sitting with her mother reinforced experiences brought over from a past life.

Often children reveal past-life habits quite early in their childhood, before the age of five. They may show an appreciation or interest in music, the arts, reading, specific activities, or scientific exploration. By encouraging their natural inclinations, you help them to develop talents from former lives. Yogananda encouraged this practice as helpful in reestablishing past good habits, reawakening talents, even finding friends from past lives. There were ten young boys born in our community within a year of one another. Most of these boys are close friends today, suggesting that they might have all chosen to come in together.

For a number of years we sang in a choir of all ages—older members mixed with young singers Rama's age. Our family would practice singing together in the car, at home, and with friends. It was one of our most positive and uplifting shared activities. The music was yogic, with encouraging messages. We'd each practice a different part, soprano or bass; until his voice changed Rama sang high tenor parts.

I recently learned the Queen of England often engaged her whole family in singing. Sometimes after dinner they'd sing along with a recording of old musicals. She also loved to dance, having learned to waltz at a young age. Pope Francis is another fan of dancing. In his book *Dear Pope Francis,* he tells children he loved to dance traditional Argentine dances and, as a young man, the tango. "You know, dancing expresses joy and happiness. When you are sad, you can't dance," he wrote. "Even the great King David danced. . . . He didn't worry about formality. He forgot to behave like a king, and he began to dance like a little child!"*

Families are supported emotionally and spiritually by special events and rituals. From the time they are born, through the age of twenty-six or even older, young people need to feel nurtured by their families and their communities. In our family, the Ananda Community and Living Wisdom Schools fulfilled some of these needs; even so the main work of raising children is left to parents. Grandparents, other family members, and close friends often help.

One practice that helped support our journey together as a family we called "holding the energy." When parents succeed in holding the energy, they are creating in their heart and their mind's eye positive energy around their children that allows the children to reach their highest potential. We try to stay true to the value system underlying the life of our own family: "In our family we do this. In our family we talk this way, we don't do things we think might hurt you or others. In our family we don't let (the media, the movies and the internet) tell us what we feel is the right thing to do. We have our own family values." By gently and honestly communicating family values, starting at a young age, we give children strength and self-confidence to know right from wrong.

---

* Pope Francis, *Dear Pope Francis* (Chicago: Loyola Press, 2016), 21.

Family values aren't normally taught in schools. Because today's young people might leave high school with no real sense of family values, American colleges are plagued with alcohol abuse, hazing, sexual abuse, even rape. Many colleges are now trying to fix this problem through orientation programs that disavow such practices. True education for life, however, begins long before we reach college, in the homes and with families.

If we see failure and fault in our children or in each other, we create a subtle thought pattern that can actually magnetize the very thing we don't want to have happen.

I had a negative experience with motorcycles when I was a teen and found myself projecting my own fears onto my family. When our son was living in New Zealand, a twenty-four-year-old friend of his was killed in a tragic motorcycle accident, an experience I'm sure shocked him. A few months after the accident, Rama announced by phone that he would rent a motorcycle and tour a bit. I could feel my blood pressure start to rise. It took all my will to relax and construct a response. I told him I loved him and cared deeply for his welfare.

One way to help others is to visualize a bubble of white light—a protective, loving light that comes from God into the heart and is channeled out to our children and family. Within the bubble include your love, positive thoughts, and positive energy. Gradually, as we deepen our own inner life, this loving energy radiates out, creating a larger energy that in an unfathomable way allows our family members to do their best. At times, I've kept a journal, writing about family experiences. At the end of six months I'd reflect on what I'd written, trying to learn and grow myself. I've learned that changing my own attitudes is a step towards greater family happiness.

Good communication skills also help family life. Many years ago I needed to communicate something very difficult to a large group of people. I asked a friend who was a therapist to help me. She introduced me to role playing. Role playing takes place between two people, usually the therapist and the client. The therapist listens carefully, then repeats back what she heard, trying to mirror the words. This process continues until the person having difficulty communicating the specific message feels confident of doing so alone.

For instance, which parent will be the one to have those talks with the daughter or son about puberty, hormones, sex, and procreation? Practicing good communication early with your partner will help. Role playing—one parent being the child, the other the parent—then switching back and forth, is one way to practice difficult discussions, and has the added benefit of bringing laughter!

Conversations that are sensitive flow more easily if you've already established good communication channels with your children—dialogues that are both respectful and loving. After the age of seven, children have a bit more reasoning ability. Once adolescence does come, which can sometimes happen sooner than we may expect, we will have in place the tools for talking about sexual activity and feelings—as well as substance abuse and peer pressure—without the children withdrawing or shutting down.

A Family Pilgrimage

A FAMILY PILGRIMAGE TOGETHER IS a way to strengthen spiritual bonds, especially if taken when the children are at an age when they can comprehend it. Finding the time and money for such a venture can take more than a year of planning, preceded of course, by lots of prayers.

When I first mentioned the idea of a family pilgrimage to Nakula, panic ran across his face. We both liked the idea but had no money for it. The pilgrimage would need to take place during the time of year when the weather was bad enough to shut down his building work. Yearning to visit Italy and the home of Saint Francis of Assisi, we began an armchair pilgrimage. We read stories to Rama about the Wolf of Gubbio (tamed by Saint Francis), listened to music about the life of Saint Francis, learned some basic Italian, and in the summer made caprese and pasta, all while keeping thoughts of a pilgrimage in the background.

By early fall we checked flight information, gauged the least expensive way to go, saved, cut corners, and prayed for guidance. The prospect of visiting our teacher, who'd recently moved to Assisi, gave us a strong incentive. In late fall it all came together. We could travel to Italy in January and stay at Ananda Europa outside Assisi on a mouse budget. Since we'd be taking

Rama out of first grade for a month, his teacher devised a project for him—to create a scrapbook of his experiences with postcards, photos, and drawings, learn eight words of Italian (and know how to spell them), and write simple sentences about some of the places he visited. To this day he remembers the experience, the scrapbook a poignant souvenir.

Each family member had pilgrimage highlights. My teacher was fluent in many languages, and especially in Italian. Our first contact with him in Italy was a talk he gave in Italian at Ananda Europa's *Tempio di Luce.* None of us really knew what he was saying. We listened with our hearts. Afterwards I felt something had shifted for me energetically. Old fears and pains were somehow being loosened; by the end of the talk I felt completely free of them.

The second gift of pilgrimage came unexpectedly. I came down with a bad cold and flu and for a few days was confined to my room. During this time one of the leaders of the Ananda Assisi community invited our family to go on an outing with my teacher into the town of Assisi. Although I was looking forward to this trip, I felt too sick to attend.

Nakula and Rama went on the outing with my teacher and I slept most of the day. While I was sleeping, the face of Yogananda appeared to me in a dream. He was looking at me and talking with me, giving me some instruction. The voice he was using was not his own voice, the voice of Yogananda, but was the voice of my teacher, Swami Kriyananda. Years later Kriyananda told me several times that he always prayed to Yogananda before he wrote or lectured, with this prayer: "Let my words be your words."

Nakula and Rama had their own pilgrimage with Swami Kriyananda that day. They toured together, shared an exquisite Italian meal, and went shopping with our teacher. They watched him closely as he lovingly greeted each shopkeeper as a best friend. His generosity and joy were contagious, with ample servings of smiles, laughter, and reveling.

Later in the month I had a long private interview with Swami Kriyananda to ask his guidance on this book about the four ashrams of life. I realize now what I could not have known then—that I was not ready spiritually to write such a book. I needed to complete my householder stage of life, raise our son, be involved with education, and live my life. He told me that the greater world wasn't ready to live in community, and explained to me the laws of magnetism. First, yogic families and others needed to live mindfully in communities, setting an example with their pioneering efforts. "In time, people will eventually just know it's more conducive to health and spiritual well-being to live in community, to live more simply, to grow their own food and help each other," he said. He spoke of a coming time when people would understand their interconnectedness with all, and the role Self-realization and Sanaatan Dharma (the "eternal religion") would play.

On our way home from Assisi, we stopped in Rome for a few days. The pope would see many hundreds of people one day each week. Nakula propped Rama up on his shoulders; they both pointed and waved at a little man standing five hundred feet away. See Rama, there's the pope. *He's a very holy person.*

Young children can be very sensitive to energy. Our son seemed okay with visiting the pope, but he did not like his experience in the Coliseum in Rome. When we walked into the Coliseum his energy began to shrink; he became somewhat fearful, even though there weren't many people around us. "This is a fighting place," he announced to us, and instantly wanted to leave. We stayed a few minutes more, then quickly left.

Many years we turned to nature for pilgrimage. We'd drive to the ocean or to a nearby campground to watch the river. In the evening we'd build a huge campfire, roast veggie dogs, and just sit. The campfire became our entertainment. We'd stare at the stars, listen to the river, do a few mantras, and put the fire to bed.

Far from the common idea of a luxury vacation, with sensory indulgence and overextended pocketbook, pilgrimage reminds us what's important on life's journey, and gives us an opportunity to share our love for and gratitude to the Divine in a much deeper way. Pilgrimage is a way to increase devotion for families.

Spiritually minded parents and caregivers soon learn how powerful are their thoughts. When we use our thoughts constructively, they become valuable tools for helping our families. Positive affirmations, which are a form of positive prayer, can be practiced along with yoga postures or after meditation to increase their effectiveness.

Of all the vibrations that exist in the universe, thoughts are the most subtle. Your thoughts can help determine your success or your failure. Being mindful of what we bring into our consciousness at bedtime helps maintain a family's peace of mind. Before retiring, consider ending each evening with family affirmations or prayers for world peace, reciting the Mahamritunjaya Mantra,* or reading something that will uplift your family's consciousness.

Prayers and Affirmations for Families

THE FOLLOWING PRAYERS ARE wonderful for invoking the positive qualities of the heart, the indwelling love, beauty, and intuitive knowledge inherent in the heart chakra. You can substitute any of the eight aspects of God (light, love, sound, peace, calmness, joy, wisdom, and power) to help focus on specific qualities to uplift our consciousness in times of need.

Once, while driving in extreme weather down a narrow mountain road above a steep river gorge, I began softly singing a chant of Yogananda's, using the word "calmness" instead of "beauty": "God of calmness is now reigning in the temple of my heart. In my heart, in my heart, in the temple of my heart." I repeated these lines over and over for several minutes. At one point I left off the words "God of calmness" and substituted a different word: "Concentration is now reigning in the temple of my heart. In my heart, in my heart, in the temple of my heart." My son said to me, "Mom, are you singing?" I answered yes, and shared with him why I was singing this chant at this particular time. The heart is the purveyor of all that is good in our consciousness. Together with the breath, the heart influences our mind and our thoughts.

Prayer for Guidance

I will reason, I will will, I will act; but guide Thou my reason, will, and activity to the right thing that I should do in everything.**

---

* See p. 54 in "Girl's Rites."

** Paramhansa Yogananda, *Whispers from Eternity* (Nevada City, California, 2008), xxi.

Prayer for Peace and Harmony

This affirmation, by Yogananda, is excellent for relationships, families, and couples, as well as for world peace. Practice after yoga or meditation, before bed, or first thing in the morning:

Repeat ten times out loud:
Lord, fill this world with peace and harmony, peace and harmony.

Repeat three times out loud:
Lord, fill me with peace and harmony, peace and harmony.

Yogananda taught a method for bringing affirmations from our conscious mind to our superconscious mind through repeating the affirmation over and over. Essential to the practice is a strong faith. Doubt weakens the will and decreases the effectiveness of your affirmations. When these affirmations are practiced correctly, over and over, they penetrate the superconscious mind and begin to affect thoughts positively. Start by saying the affirmation loudly and affirmatively. Next, repeat the affirmation in your normal speaking voice. Then, repeat the affirmation in a whisper. Finally, focusing at the spiritual eye (the point between the eyebrows which Yogananda called the "Christ Center"), repeat the affirmation mentally.

Affirmation for Psychological Success

Yogananda's psychological success affirmation, from *Scientific Healing Affirmations*, can be practiced several times a day. Many people have been helped by this affirmation. Nakula told me he used it when he was a young man wanting to bring more success and prosperity into his life. He recorded himself saying the affirmation then played it over and over when he was driving. After six months his life began to turn around in many positive ways.

I am brave, I am strong.
Perfume of success thought
Blows in me, blows in me.
I am cool, I am calm
I am sweet, I am kind

Family Yoga

I am love, I am sympathy
I am charming and magnetic
I am pleased with all
I wipe the tears and fears of all
I have no enemy
Though some think they are so.
I am the friend of all.
I have no habits,
In eating, thinking, behaving
I am free, I am free.

I command Thee, O Attention
To come and practice concentration
On things I do, on works I do.
I can do everything
When so I think, when so I think.

In church or temple, in prayer mood
My vagrant thoughts against me stood
And held my mind from reaching Thee
And held my mind from reaching Thee
Teach me to own again, O own again
My matter-sold mind and brain
That I may give them to Thee
In prayer and ecstasy
In meditation and reverie.

I shall worship Thee
In meditation
In the mountain breast and seclusion.
I shall feel Thy energy
Flowing through my hands in activity
Lest I lose Thee
I shall find Thee in activity.*

---

* From *Scientific Healing Affirmations* by Paramhansa Yogananda, 1924 edition.

There are many affirmations for attracting positive results and keeping the mind uplifted. Here is one from *Affirmations for Self-Healing* on success.

Success

True success means transcendence. It means finding what we really want, which is not outward things, but inner peace of mind, self-understanding—and, above all, the joy of God.

Outward success means transcendence also. It means rising above past accomplishments to reach new levels of achievement. Success can mean accepting failure, too, when such acceptance helps us to transcend a false ambition. Every failure, moreover, can be a steppingstone to highest achievement.

Success should not be measured by the things accomplished, but by our increasing understanding, ability, and closeness to God.

Affirmation

I leave behind me both my failures and accomplishments. What I do today will create a new and better future, filled with inner joy.

Prayer

O Creator of galaxies and countless, blazing stars, the power of the very universe is Thine! May I reflect that power in the little mirror of my life and consciousness.[*]

* Swami Kriyananda, *Affirmations for Self Healing* (Nevada City, California: Crystal Clarity Publishers, 2005), 20–21.

CHAPTER 14

Brahmachari Aditya

WHEN ADITYA WAS TWENTY-FOUR, he was very close to marriage. He and his prospective wife were both medical students, studying to become doctors, and she was a wonderful girl. "When we were together, I remember asking her how she felt about serving together as doctors in a rural area. She was not interested, and for me something shifted. I always wanted to serve in a rural area of India."

From the time he was in sixth grade he had wanted to become a doctor. "People's pain has always moved me," he explained. "I always wanted to be a doctor because I wanted to help people." Born in Rajasthan, he attended schools in Pune, then Lucknow, Alwar, and Visakhaptnam in Andra Pradesh, then back to Pune for medical studies, finally doing his residency in surgery at St. Stephen's Hospital in Delhi.

Born and raised in India, Aditya read extensively about the life of Gandhi, popularly considered to be the father of the nation of India. "I had wondered if there was someone who had a solution for the world's problems," he said. "I knew if I kept thinking about these solutions on my own I'd go crazy. There were no solutions in the media, from politicians, even from the religious leaders in our country. I knew Gandhi had had a spiritual practice. I was searching."

"It was around this time that I found *Autobiography of a Yogi* in a Delhi bookstore. When I read the book, it was clear to me that Yogananda knew the way out. So I filled out the postcard inside the book for more information, but no one ever contacted me. Three weeks later I saw an ad with Yogananda's photo with that of Swami Kriyananda." There was a glow that came from the two photos. "I went to hear one of Swamiji's talks. He was elderly, and I remembered nothing of what he said, but the moment I saw him I knew that he had absorbed all of Yogananda's teachings.

"He was sitting in a chair, and I was watching his eyes. I had only two or three seconds of darshan with him. I could tell even from this brief meeting how frail he was." Deeper than the frail body, Aditya felt Kriyananda's profound sincerity and devotion to his guru. "What I saw and felt was a lifetime of teachings, so I wrote him a letter," he explained. In his letter, Aditya told Swami Kriyananda that he was a doctor, and that he'd taken care of orphans, the elderly, all sorts of people. "If you think I'd be any use in your organization, I'd like to help," he offered.

"I wanted an interview with the swami. I began praying to Yogananda and to Kriyananda. I kept my prayers up for eighteen months. Even though I was practicing medicine, I knew what I was doing wasn't the highest for myself. The thought occurred to me, *What if he calls me? Would I really be able to do what he wanted me to do?*"

"I was serving in a rural hospital near Delhi. I had just finished fifty hours of service, including three caesarian sections. My energy was so high I felt I could have done five more. Although people at the hospital were congratulating me, I was thinking, *This is nothing.* I went home, looked at the book I'd been reading, and said to the photo, 'I could do more, much more. But if I ever come to you, you should have much more work for me to do.'

"I was getting a response: *It's going to happen soon.*" On an inner level, Aditya felt he was being tested. "Very soon after those surgeries, and soon after my experience of 'talking with the book,' I called the Ananda Center near Delhi, asking to meet with Swamiji in October 2008. I had realized that I had been relying on the guru coming to the disciple, rather than the disciple going to the guru." When Aditya called for an interview, Swami was still in America, not to return until November. "On November 22 I went to a talk he was giving called Hope for a Better World. *That's* what I wanted. There were seven hundred people there, and I could not even get close to him."

"That night I put aside all my fears. *Aren't you sure in yourself about your search for God?*, I was asking myself. Four days later I went to the Ananda Sangha ashram in Gurgaon, and attended their satsang. There were many people there, and several of them were asking Swami questions. I started to ask a question, but before I could finish asking, Swami answered, 'Man's highest responsibility in this life is to find God, and I think you did the right thing by coming here.' That was it. He was answering the question I had asked him in my letter.

"Later, when I first met him he said to me, 'What do you think of starting a rural hospital at our community in Pune?' Swami knew I wanted to become a monk, and so he gave me my vows. Since taking my vows I have become Yogananda's own. Not once have I thought about dropping the vows. For me, what's important is tuning in to my Guru and doing his will through the living instrument of this body. Yes, my parents were disappointed—especially my father, a doctor himself. Now, many years since my first taking vows, they respect what I'm doing.

"I'm very practical. I meet many people, so it's very helpful that I'm a doctor. I talk to corporations, leaders, and businesspeople. I'm sharing the practical and health benefits of yoga and the teachings I follow. I help people with stress management, obesity, diet, insomnia, hypertension, overcoming fatigue—any number of ailments. One man, about sixty years of age, told me he used to pray every day and thank God for everything. He used to walk to a lake near his village and watch the sunset. He would pray and thank God for everything. 'But,' then he would say, 'why God, did you give me this pain?' He had trauma to his knees and legs, trauma which also affected his back. I spent seven or eight minutes with him. I taught him some unique exercises and the full yogic breath, with tension and relaxation. He practiced what I taught him, and healed himself. He comes back, and he thanks me for helping him. He can walk without pain, and now has no pain in his legs, knees, or back.

"Monastic life is one of selfless service. It's a very direct path of selflessness, devotion, loyalty to one's teacher, and living a life of high ideals. It's also a life of deep contentment. In giving everything of oneself comes a joyful, expansive inner freedom."

I asked him about brahmacharya as discipline: "Do you feel an overarching theme of discipline in your life?" "It's a life of service," Aditya replied. "The more I think of others, the fewer problems arise within myself. A monk who is selfish is going to have a terrible life.

"The small self or the large Self, which are you going to choose? When I choose the large Self," Aditya concluded, "it's effortless—no discipline is required."

CHAPTER 15

*"May the longtime sun shine upon you, all love surround you, and
the pure light within you, guide your way on."*

—Celtic song performed after practicing
Yogi Bhajan's Kundalini Yoga

Nefretete

"YOU'VE SEEN THE MOVIE *Birdman?*" she inquired. I shook my head. "I know what it's about, but I haven't seen it," I answered. "Well, that's what my life was like with the New York theatre world." She chuckled and laughed, then chuckled again. "Picking people off the walls, the whole crazy thing. It was a lot like the movie portrayed. There were many wonderful times too, but I feel like I have finished that karma."

It was 1980 and Nefretete Rasheed was heading for New York City after graduating from Howard University in Washington, D.C. She was very organized. "I had a job and a place to live before moving there. I was doing office work for a lieutenant major in the Salvation Army and on the side I was dancing eight to ten hours a day, sometimes later into the night."

Because the studios were all centrally located in New York, travel to auditioning and training became easy. She worked and trained with such dancers as Merce Cunningham, Martha Graham, and Alvin Ailey, auditioned side-by-side with well-known actors, and was constantly looking for work as an actress/singer.

"Every day was a day at the carnival." Nefretete smiled. "In New York, you're always on to your next thing. I was in full-forward drive for fifteen of the twenty-five years I lived there. People in theatre are so hungry for work they'll do almost anything to get it. So many things are pulling on you all at the same time that it takes everything you have to hold onto yourself and keep your center.

Her training as a writer also helped her career. "I worked at The Public Theater with Joe Papp, who at the time was one of the hottest producers. I remember meeting with him at the theater, then rushing uptown to have another meeting with Alvin Ailey and one of my teachers. I was having a good time. I ended up working with a lot of different productions and with a lot of gifted and wonderful people." As her reputation grew, she was involved in more and more productions—not just in New York, but all over the world. She eventually became assistant director for one of the programs at Joseph Papp's New York Shakespeare Festival.

"I always had my suitcase packed and ready to go," she remembered. "There was always an adventure. We did shows in Italy, Africa, the Caribbean, Europe, Paris, Germany, Switzerland, and Australia."

"Did these experiences change you?" I asked her. "I had feelings of how precarious, ephemeral, and unreal it all was," she answered. "I'd be in an audition with someone I'd seen in the movies when I was younger, and I'd inwardly ask, 'You *still have to come down here and audition?*'" "What would happen to people?" I asked. "They would get stuck, and sometimes they'd get a little crazy. They were afraid. It was often a risky business."

She referred me to a show on Netflix called *House of Cards,* which won several awards. "You watch that show and see what extremes people will go to just to hang on to their power." She continued, "People sometimes go to extremes in the theatre. You always had to remain flexible and creative; my need was to be very unattached. You always had to be ready for the next thing. Without my little day planner I would have been lost. And the great expense of living in New York kept you constantly on your toes, moving forward."

"So what changed for you?" I asked her. "I was backstage in the dressing room one night, keeping everyone calm before a performance. There were some very talented actors—veterans, we called them—who'd been in theater a long time. You know, they'd spend six hours just working on one word of their lines," she sighed. "I remember thinking I wasn't sure I wanted to spend twenty more years at this." She paused and looked at me, "'I'm just passing through' was my motto. I told myself, 'I'm only doing this for a few more years.' I'd been involved for nearly fifteen years at that point. I had gone back to school to get my MA in Literature and Writing and my PhD in Psychology and Drama Therapy.

"Anyway, one day I was backstage before a dance program, and I overheard someone say something about a 'sweat,'" she said. "You mean a sweat lodge?" I asked her. "No, I just heard talk about a sweat. It was some sort of Native American ceremony. One of the women urged me to go to the Native American empowerment circle. Something inside me said, *Yeah, you should go.*"

"Where was the sweat?" I asked her. "The sweats were in upstate New York, and you know how beautiful it is up there," she said. "The fall colors, the trees and mountains—they were calling to me. The group was led by a Lakota chief who owned thousands of acres down the Baja in Mexico at a place called Los Dolores. I became very involved. We used to go down there to perform a traditional Lakota Ceremony called Spirit Dance. We'd go in early November, and from midnight to dawn, we'd dance on top of the mountain under the stars. The land was eight hours by boat from La Paz. There were no paved roads. It was pristine and untouched, nothing there but mountains and water.

"The ocean was crystal clear and the dolphins would swim alongside our boat. We saw whales and beautiful tropical fish. There had once been a monastery at Los Dolores. Remnants of a vineyard were still there a couple of miles inland from the beach. It was exquisitely beautiful.

"Decades ago the chief and his wife were sent to the States by their guru to lead an ashram in Minnesota, and later to teach yoga to the Native Americans. Suffice it to say they picked up the Native American traditions and ultimately assumed tremendous responsibilities as keepers of the Lakota traditions. They established a community and an esoteric school that fused both

Native American traditions and Eastern traditions. Years later, I became one of the directors for the upstate school.

"The chief and his wife spent many years in upstate New York and developed a community of pipe carriers, students, and adherents. They conducted traditional sweat lodges and performed many services for the community through the men's and women's councils they established. We had many duties, responsibilities, and disciplines to maintain and observe. I never had an interest in becoming a pipe carrier because I knew it was not my path, but I was honored to be invited to travel with them to the Sun Dance ceremonies at the reservation in South Dakota, and to Spirit Dance in Mexico. I was at the same time very passionate about spiritual studies and practices. We studied yoga, comparative religion, astrology, the chakras, Hermetic philosophy, and much more. It was with this group of people that I participated in and later taught empowerment courses in New York City.

"So this is the long story of how I stayed connected to yoga and spiritual practice I had begun as a teenager. I did a Vision Quest with the chief around 1996—four days and nights alone in the woods of upstate New York with a prayer for myself to find and follow a spiritual path. At the time I had no idea what that path was. Another decade would pass before I fully understood what I was praying for in those woods. These ceremonies and the Vision Quest were peak and transformative experiences—it's difficult for me to find words to explain."

I asked Nefretete about her youth. From the time she was a young girl, she had a profound inner life, one the adults surrounding her were completely unaware of. "Adults always like to think they can keep things from kids. We're not supposed to know what they know." She laughed and smiled. "I was a young, very sensitive African-American girl growing up in Washington, D.C. in the seventies. Nothing quite made sense to me. I wanted to be an astronomer; I was artistic and creative. I knew there was something more to life. When I was about twelve, I remember watching Richard Hittleman doing yoga on television—a window into another world."

She told me she loved nature and wasn't all that interested in playing with dolls. "It just didn't look like fun. I had already sensed I didn't want to have kids. Washington, D.C. can be very conservative. I had a very stable life in the Episcopalian church that my family belonged to. At the same time, I really enjoyed going to the African Methodist Episcopal [AME] church with some of my friends. The AME church was fun and not so stuffy. They had bible school, cupcakes, and an amazing choir. The music was very lively and magnetic. It did something for my heart—I could feel the power of Jesus, and I knew he loved me.

"For me, The Ebony Impromptu Theater Company, which was an African-American theatre group, was my first community. We all did Transcendental Meditation and became vegetarians together. We met several times a week. The group became a second family to me.

"As an artist, you're naturally creative, and you learn to move to the side and let things move through you. I felt my parents didn't really know me. It was the arts that saved me. Although my first creative focus had been the visual arts, now I left my paint brushes behind and fell in love with the energy, fun, and adventure of theatre. Theatre fit my spirit."

In her senior year in high school and beginning years in college, the camaraderie of the theatre group brought something unexpected.

"One night, we all decided to do a séance together. Although our theatre director didn't like us doing a séance, he agreed that could do it *one* time, but never again. We sat in a circle and prayed. Nothing happened. Something *had* happened, but we weren't aware of it. The theatre group was intergenerational, of all ages. A ten-year-old boy was taking part in the séance. He saw something appear and told the group what it was. Things started happening. Someone called in the spirit of Paul Robeson, the famous African-American singer and actor who sang 'Old Man River'—and one of the first black men to perform Othello on stage.

"His spirit was so huge that I could feel it. But I also felt that I became his joy and laughter. Later, I felt I'd become other aspects of his consciousness, including a sadness. When someone asked him, 'What is success?' he just laughed. For me, to feel that much energy was a powerful experience. I could feel the energy in my spine. I had passed out of my body. It was a very joyful experience. I could feel that I was out of my body.

"During the séance a realization came to me: 'It's love that brought you here to this earth plane, and it's love that keeps you here.' I understood that we're really just channels for what's going on, for the energy that is in us and all around us. My whole life I'd been trying to figure out what's going on. After that experience, I knew there was something much more. Finally, I had concrete proof of what I'd long suspected.

"When I was seventeen, while practicing Kundalini Yoga, I had another out-of-body experience. The class was lying down in the Savasana pose. I remember the chanting, and the words: 'May the longtime sun shine upon you, all love surround you, and the pure light within you, guide your way on.' The lyrics come from an old Celtic tune. When Yogi Bhajan heard this song, he instructed his students to sing it at the end of every yoga class they taught.

"We also sang *Ek Ong Kar Sat Nam Siri Wahe Guru,*" from the Gurmukhi language: 'The Creator and Creation are One; this is our True Identity; the ecstasy of the experience of this wisdom is beyond all words and brings indescribable bliss.' Here was the first mantra taught by Yogi Bhajan in the United States—what he called the mantra of the Aquarian Age.

"After my first out-of-body experience doing yoga, I remember leaving the ashram house and walking down the street with a couple of my friends from the theater company. Everything was shimmering and glistening. Buckets of silver and golden light seemed to be pouring out over everything. Everything vibrated. I felt electric. My feet seemed not to be touching the ground. I felt ecstatic—full of energy and light.

"Before this experience I had had no idea who the Sikhs were or who Yogi Bhajan really was—just that he was deeply respected. Everyone seemed to scurry about when he was approaching or present. He and his followers had a couple of stores in Georgetown, and, on Connecticut Avenue, my favorite restaurant, The Golden Temple. There were hardly any vegetarian places around at that time. I did not feel strongly compelled to become a Sikh and wear those beautiful white clothes—it was bizarre enough for my family that I was an artist kid who had cut her hair off and wrapped it up in geles and wore long earrings, long dresses, and bangles. These experiences were a beginning, a serious confirmation that I was on the right road in my search for the truth of things."

CHAPTER 16

The Veil

IT WAS ONE OF those late afternoons when pale blue skies turn shades of rose petal. We boarded our car, bumped down the steep access from the Meditation Retreat, maneuvered through dirt and gravel, the road still littered with pine needles and broken limbs from a rousing storm.

We passed the 'Inimim, an old growth forest our neighbors were helping to preserve. Earlier in the year, we worked together to remove underbrush from the big trees protected there. The result has been happier neighbors and healthier lives. Today, as we drove through the forest, something dark moved above and before us.

"There he is," my husband sang, "Nevermore, nevermore!" Our eyes looked up. The raven, symbol of magic and messenger between worlds, darted high in front of the car, as he often did, piloting us through the forest. We live where the Nisenan roamed hundreds of years before; I feel their hand whenever these birds fly into our lives. Poe's Raven sang to us. *Nevermore, nevermore, nevermore can we keep the love of mortals; life will always give us gains and losses.*

As we continued, the late afternoon light made the corridor seem murky and closed-in; the Manzanita reached for our car; the pines held a steep salute; the trees weave a story. We traveled the Trail of the Blissful Burro, renamed for its predecessor, Jackass Flats. Then down through another forest corridor opening to a wide and barren landscape. Early days of gold mining had left remnants, ravaged piles of falling topsoil, stunted trees. Water cannons had divided the earth in search for gold. A moonscape remained.

Greed had inspired the destruction, wiping out Nisenan trails, building a new history. I tried to imagine the Nisenan living simply, the land their own mother. When we reached the pavement our old car sighed. Now we sped through taller forests, up and down a rollercoaster, the road sleek, scenic, carrying us faster. Another raven wove out in front, flying faster to keep in front of us. My husband remarked that it must be his spirit guide.

We made the turn into Ananda Village, moved through the valley, then up the long hill to one of the highest points on the land. I remembered my first coming here when all the roads were dirt. During the rains the dust and orange clay would turn to peanut-butter consistency, cars would sink in the mud. Pavement became our desire. We descended quickly towards our destination: an abrupt ledge overlooking steep canyons. Below, the Middle Fork of the Yuba River was hiding, crawling.

Hand-in-hand we continued in silence towards the meeting. The carved wooden gates opened softly. We floated onto a scenic verandah with statues, chimes, a Mediterranean-style building that welcomed us. Other couples gathered. We descended farther down steps, riding the crest from above.

To our left a pool bubbled before a resilient Quan Yin, her eyes downcast, fingers holding skirts in a modest bow, elegantly androgynous. She seemed transported from another world to greet the yogi couples.

Halfway down the steep stairs we were forced to pause, stepping out onto a lush terrace bordered by shrubbery. We gazed into the vast expanse. The sky seemed touchable, a painted set from an epic film. Forested hills wove up and down the steep canyon, mountains in the distance. We walked to the edge and peeked over the side. One thousand feet below, a serpent of rock and water moved westward. Holding completely still, we listened for its sound. More silence. Was it the water that was singing as it rushed onward?

We turned and continued our journey down, past the storybook chapel and tiered gardens so artistically painted just for us. Beyond was a huge domed building surrounded by more gardens, a stoic Buddha in meditation pose standing guard.

We walked into the dome, the heart of the Crystal Hermitage. Couples were gathering, shyly waiting. Statues of saints "hovered" near the altar. Beyond the windows stood a view that was distractingly expansive. Candles were lit, the light casting an ethereal glow towards the woodlands that lay beyond.

Most of the couples knew each other, and smiled warmly. There were old couples, middle-aged couples, young couples. Most were dressed in white, those who had taken final vows in blue. Community leaders Jyotish and Devi welcomed us. "We will all renew our marriage vows together," Devi said. "Let us usher in a new era for married renunciates to offer the world a yogic model of spiritual marriage," she added quietly. Jyotish offered a prayer. We chanted softly, then meditated.

Opening my eyes afterwards, I noticed the room had darkened, candles seemed brighter in the early evening light. There was a feeling of anticipation. The time came to begin the long wedding vow renewal ceremony. Couples faced each other, locked eyes, and repeated the vows as Jyotish and Devi read them.

I remembered our wedding day. Was I really getting married? I remember turning twenty-four and thinking that I would *never* get married, that marriage just wasn't something I would do. More than twenty-four years had passed and here we stood, as if it were yesterday.

"I will merge the opposites of duality," we repeated to each other. And my favorite line, "May our love grow ever stronger, deeper, more expansive, until in our perfected love we find the perfect love of God."

I caught a glimpse of couples holding hands, smiling like newlyweds. The trees were our audience. The darkening sky waved. The vow renewal was over. We were planting seeds.

After the ceremony some remained, laughing and congratulating each other. We walked out to catch the first stars. A marriage ritual is the natural affirmation for couples walking the householder path together.

Renewing wedding vows each year reminds us why we married; it allows us to take a deeper step together and serves as way to be purified and blessed for the next stage of our journey. Weddings naturally involve heart energy, an abundance of love flowing to each other and out to the world. Choosing to renew vows with others can be a service that is stabilizing, lending support, magnetism, and love to couples who may be secretly struggling.

Holy Vows at Marriage

(Expressed first by the couple to God.)

Beloved Lord,
We dedicate to Thee our lives, our service, and the love we share.
May the communion we find with one another lead us to inner communion with Thee.
May the service we render one another perfect in us our service of Thee.
May we behold Thee always enshrined in one another's forms.
May we always remember that it is above all Thee we love.

In every test of love, may we see Thy loving hand.
In every disagreement, may we seek Thy hidden guidance.
May our love not be confined by selfish needs.
     but give us the strength ever to expand our hearts
      until we see all human beings, all creatures as our own.
Teach us to love all beings equally, in Thee.

(The couple then speaks these vows to each other.)

Dear Beloved,
I will be true to you as I pray always to be true to God.
I will love you without condition, as I would be loved
     by you—and as we are ever loved by God.
I will never compete with you; I will cooperate for our own,
     and for all others', highest good.
I will forgive you always, and under all circumstances.
I will respect your right to see truth as you perceive it,
     and to be guided as you feel deeply within yourself,
     and I will work with you always, in freedom,
     to arrive at a common understanding.

All that we do, may we do for God's glory.
May we live and grow together in His love and joy.

And may the offspring of our union—
      whether human children or creative deeds—
      be doorways for the inspiration that we feel from Him,
      through each other.
May our love grow ever deeper, purer, more expansive,
      until, in our perfected love,
      we find the perfect love of God.*

---

* Ananda Wedding Vows, as published in *Self-Expansion Through Marriage* by Swami Kri-yananda (Nevada City, California: Crystal Clarity Publishers, 1995), 162–64.

CHAPTER 17

Premabhava

This fiction story explores the astral realms of Premabhava.

ON A DISTANT GALAXY there exists an astral heaven so subtle its very existence can only be seen through yogic vision. Souls drawn here are mainly characterized by their most recent relationships on earth. These liaisons may have ended abruptly or with deep sadness. Perhaps two souls have been family members, close friends, or lovers, but somehow through the inevitability that is life, one or the other fell into longing and grief.

This planet is called Premabhava, known as "the feeling of love." Among the millions of heavenly abodes, it is an astral region offering a specific kind of healing. Some come here to cure their grief. Others come to drink from the ether of a love they have long lost touch with.

If there has been extreme disharmony between two souls bound by matrimony, Premabhava served as a hermitage within which to reconnect with qualities of love that exist deep within each soul. For grief-stricken souls for whom an early or abrupt departure from earth seem unfounded, Premabhava offers a celebration of the highest attainments that earthly love can express for two individual souls. Through deep intuition and soul desire, yogis can travel here.

The entrance to Premabhava is veiled behind a lustrous white canyon of clouds that shift with gentle winds. As the traveler enters, amethyst light beckons like a giant sea anemone, pulsating and churning. A tranquil ocean surrounded by steep white cliffs invites the travelers to gaze into its waters.

Nearby, a seaside village lounges on the riviera. Birds dive and spin through clouds, guiding visitors. An odd species of lavender birds circle and swirl, long golden beaks emitting sounds like tiny chimes. Dancers emerge appareled in lotus-colored gauze, ankles sprinkled with bells that flash as they leap and twirl across the scene. From a steep mountain of azure fog comes the steady rhythm of a temple gong, a salve that heals the heart. Across the forest an alto chime responds.

Beyond the valley a motherly figure appears, a harpsichord clasped to her breast. She gazes at each visitor through a large singular open eye, situated above and between two closed eyes. Her thoughts seem lost in a distant language few remember. The bell sounds that emerge from her instrument cause souls to stop and listen for what may seem eternity.

When the motherly figure stops playing, crystalline sprites arrive at her side. Merrily hoisting the instrument atop their heads, they dance and spin away through the mist. Gazing into the very heart of the soul in front of her, the Divine Being begins to sing. She serenades each visitor with a voice no human could begin to imitate. It is an intimate love song, created to mirror the longings hidden in each soul. Often her astral tears form, and as they fall, morph into a symphony uniquely designed for each visitor. In Premabhava it is easy to forget the earth world.

FAR AWAY, IN A hill town in Italy on planet Earth lived a young woman who was caged in a body so malformed she hid it beneath a flowing cloak. She carried with her a large flowered basket of exotic breads. Some breads were twisted into braids, others were decorated with a medley of seeds and nuts. A few she filled with delicate sweet creams.

Her name was Chiara and, though she was twenty-four years old, she lived with her aunt and uncle in the country outside the village. Her life was simple and quiet.

When Chiara visited the village, she would move through crowds of merchants, scurrying along the cobbled streets as though she were floating in the sky— for she had discovered that the only way to hide her deformity was to appear as though her body were not there at all.

In a narrow corridor off a sunny street lived a family with two handsome and likeable sons. The family owned a café people from all over had come to appreciate. The two sons ran the café and had learned to create menus that were irresistible. There were asparagus bisques; vegetable terrines in puff pastry; salads with arugula, pine nuts, chevre, and nectarines; desserts of tiramisu; and elegant cups of cappuccino.

The practical son was named Antonio. Devoted, hardworking, and handsome, he was always able to recognize a bargain and help his family business become more successful. The other son, Piero, also worked hard. Piero was one of the most charming young men in the village. His eyes could melt those of strangers, and he was never at a loss for companionship.

Chiara delivered her home-baked breads to the café run by the two sons. From the moment she met Piero she felt a deep yearning in her heart and longed to be close to him. She became so filled with feelings of love when she saw Piero that she began to transfer that love into the breads she made.

When she went home each afternoon she would sing and create bread as though she were an artist painting the Italian countryside. First, she would find an exquisite combination of seeds and set them aside in small bowls. Then, before beginning, she would offer a song to those who would eat her bread. Throughout the entire ritual she would pour her heart's love into the bread.

Chiara also cast into her bread her longing for a companion who would soothe her heart and share her simple life.

It was no secret that Chiara's fanciful breads were the highlight of Antonio and Piero's café. Each morning when Piero would have his toast, he would select a piece from Chiara's breadbasket. Both he and Antonio felt Chiara had the best recipe in the entire village.

As the years wore on, the two sons married. Their wives were young and lovely and physically attractive. They bore children for the two sons, and their families worked together in the café, which now had grown larger and more famous.

Chiara's life had changed too. When Piero met his young wife his life became so absorbed with his wife's world that he stopped noticing the young girl who sold bread to the café.

Feeling more alone now, less inspired in her baking, Chiara struggled to keep love flowing into her bread.

As time moved on Antonio became the manager of the café, and his practical nature continued to help the families of both brothers. Over the years, by a strange twist of fate, Piero became disenchanted with his life, his family, and his work. He longed for a life he couldn't describe; his marriage fell apart, and with it so did his enthusiasm for work and his affection for his children. His wife left him, and, after several years of separation, found a new partner and began a new marriage, one that promised to be happy.

Piero began to wander the countryside and eventually found solace with a small group of monks who had given their lives to God. Slowly, recovering from a painfully broken heart, Piero began to change. Things like money and a home that once had seemed important to him no longer seemed necessary. He began to smile more. Piero became known as "the smiling monk," and his smiles offered warmth to many a lonely soul.

As he aged, Piero suffered from a disease that ravaged his body and his mind. The monks cared for him and would often sing to him as he rested in his bed. One day, when it became clear Piero didn't have much longer to live, a strange woman came to the small hermitage.

She was an old woman and covered in flowing capes. It was Chiara. The years had not been easy on her. As she walked towards the door, she struggled with her leg, yet in her arms she carried a most beautiful basket of decorated breads. The monks invited her inside.

She walked into the room where Piero lay in his bed. She knelt down beside him, not knowing who he was. With her head bowed in a silent prayer, she reached into her basket and pulled out an elegant roll topped with intricate seeds of all shapes and sizes. As she handed the roll to Piero, their eyes met. Though Piero had seen the young girl decades ago, he had never truly looked into her eyes. Piero blinked and gazed at the flowing robes with their misshapen outlines. He held the roll and examined it. It felt like a tiny jeweled crown. Not knowing what to say, he looked again at Chiara.

Chiara felt a feather stir in the region of her heart. As they drank in the meaning of this simple exchange, the room fell into silence. Something like a flame that burned in the heart of Piero also burned in the heart of Chiara, and for a few seconds the two flames tried to reach out to each other.

Then two heavenly flames emerged like floating kites from the soul of Piero and the soul of Chiara. What happened next went so quickly that neither could believe it was not a dream. The floating lights that had come out of their bodies merged into one flame that disappeared back into the two bodies—the body of Piero and the body of Chiara.

The beauty of the two flames merging transformed the small room. Made whole by the completeness of their love, each one's smile became the other's smile; they knew everything about each other. Never before in their millions of human lives had they experienced such feelings. They were instantly aware of each other's thoughts and began to communicate as one soul. For several moments they held hands and saw through their eyes the subtle meaning of this miraculous interchange.

After several minutes it was time to part. Chiara and Piero each knew their lives would move on in different directions. Chiara returned to her bread making. Piero sewed love into each smile he shared with the many disenfranchised souls he comforted. People would come from all over to the hermitage just to spend time at his bedside. His heart was no longer lonely, but now full with love for every living thing. Chiara's loneliness also was gone, and in its place was a heart flowing with a newfound sense of spiritual completion. Into her bread she now cast such love and completeness that some were healed even as they held a morsel.

Both knew their time on earth was nearing its end. Piero left his body first. His disease had destroyed his ability to walk and feel, and though he occasionally had visitors, his memory had long since vanished. Chiara knew instantly when Piero went; she had felt it coming for several weeks. After his passing, she wept for days; occasionally a tear would run down her face onto the bread she lovingly continued to knead, decorate, and bake.

In times of deepest silence and meditation, the two souls often communicated with each other. Although Piero tried to share with Chiara the freedom and love he was experiencing without his failing body, her grief did not lessen. Within a few months Chiara's body began to fail her, and her world started to dissolve. She longed to know the freedom Piero was experiencing, but was somehow held back.

When, years later, Chiara herself passed, her soul and astral body floated to a higher plane so refined that the heavenly devas created a ceremony just for her. Bright stars heralded her ascent, and a parade of angels, dancers, and musicians welcomed her into a deep peace.

She saw before her a tranquil sea surrounded by steep white cliffs. Gazing silently into the water, she reflected on her life and felt uplifted. Then her eye caught sight of a small Italian village, resting peacefully on a riviera. By the power of her thoughts she moved to the village, then wandered the streets. They reminded her of the Isle of Capri, a place she had once longed to visit in Italy, but had only read about.

She visited an artist's gallery, stopped at a clothing store, and admired the blooms of an elder's flower shop. The woman looked familiar; they smiled and waved to each other.

Then Chiara caught her own reflection in a shop window. A young girl of around twenty-four years smiled back at her. She had long black hair and was dressed in a perfect body, all handicaps gone. Chiara looked down at herself, feeling relieved to be out of her earthly body.

At last she arrived at an enticing café, situated on a cliff overlooking the turquoise sea. It looked like a fairy tale cottage with flower boxes filled with bright geraniums. She opened a baby-blue-colored door and walked in.

Sitting at a large round table were all her friends and family, and those she held most dear. There were her aunt and uncle, who smiled and hugged her, laughing with joy. There was her friend Cecilia, and many others. Out from under the table peeked Theodore, the dachshund she had once loved so much. At the end of the table sat a young Saint Francis, dressed in his brown robes. He rose, bowed silently, then looked into her eyes. She looked down. There, sitting on the floor next to Francis was the Wolf of Gubbio, grinning at her like a big happy dog, tongue and tail both wagging. Chiara reached down to pet the wolf and received in return a loving lick on her cheek.

She noticed the table was covered with floral china plates and cups filled with steaming cappuccino. On each plate was delicate pastry filled with exotic sweet creams. As her friends sampled the pastries they thanked her many times over, laughing and smiling. They laughed so much that even she began to laugh and smile. It was just as she had always hoped it would be.

Saint Francis moved next to her, whispered something that led to an intense discussion. Then they both smiled and laughed. Chiara spent a little more time with her family and friends, then she began her journey to Prem-abhava Mountain.

Following her inner guidance, she found the lavender birds that led her to the snow-covered peaks and steep forests Saint Francis had described to her. She saw swirling clouds and pulsating sea anemone colors. A gentle amethyst rain fell from the sky, and tiny emerald gems occasionally landed on her hands. The clouds called to her.

As she flew into their comforting vibrations she felt the presence of a familiar entity. A motherly figure emerged from clouds of pink fluorite. As the motherly figure looked into Chiara's soul, Chiara began to remember this presence, but with a difference. The motherly figure was both father and mother. She looked again. Before her stood the astral body of Piero himself, transformed into a heavenly androgynous being, beyond comprehension. As he embraced her, Chiara began to merge into his form, the two becoming one. It was the culmination of their meeting on earth, a mystic embrace of unspeakable bliss, one that she needed for the last stage of her journey to enlightenment.

∽

THE STORY OF PIERO and Chiara is a story of twin flames. In relationships, two souls become attracted to each other often because one offers something the other needs for inner completion. Twin flames is a concept Yogananda rarely talked about, and then only in the context of something each soul needed to do before achieving final liberation from the cycle of reincarnation.

My teacher also spoke of twin flames, saying there must be at least one contact with your twin soul before enlightenment. This contact needn't be of a romantic or sexual nature; it may not even be with a person of the opposite sex. The contact can be between two friends or even casual acquaintances. Your twin soul may be here on earth or even on another planet. The contact may not take place in this particular lifetime; it can even happen in a vision. Because of the intricacy of the web of karma and reincarnation, little is known about how and when twin flames reunite. Eventually though, when the time is spiritually right, it will take place without your having to search for it. You will just know.

Twin flames start out as one flame; the one flame splits into two flames, each residing in a unique body. Your twin flame is not so much the other half of your soul, as a holding pattern of various feminine and masculine energies that, when merged with your own, provide the balance needed for both individual souls to become enlightened. All relationships in life are stepping-stones to union or *yoga* with the twin flame.

My teacher once told an audience that the reason Yoganananda seldom spoke about twin flames was that the concept could easily be misinterpreted. "Because," my teacher said, "people end up thinking that every time they see anybody on a street corner, it's got to be their soul mate; and every pleasant conversation in a bar-room is with their soul mate."

Though soul-mate relationships can certainly happen, the truth behind them is deeply impersonal. From within comes the longing in our hearts for love and companionship, perhaps the greatest longing we will ever have. In a child we may see this longing fulfilled with a stuffed animal or a pet. It is born from the simple reality that it is human nature to share love. Each soul is like a tiny flame, part of a huge universal flame calling us to merge back into itself. The love for each other, and the love given us by our Creator, are one and the same.

CHAPTER 18

The Forest Dweller—Age 48–72

IN VEDIC LORE THE conch shell is a symbol.

Arjuna, the hero of India's epic Mahabharata, blew a particularly powerful conch as a battle horn. It was said to banish evil spirits, avert natural disasters, and scare away poisonous creatures. The conch is a symbol for the breath. Breath controls mind, and when the breath is correct it allows us to reach more and more blissful and higher states of samadhi.

The third stage of yoga brings us face to face with the reality of the Forest Dweller; we are finally able to examine our life for its true purpose—to develop our latent spiritual gifts even as we gradually withdraw from the world.

Just as the conch spirals in a clockwise direction—signifying expansion, eternity, and continually evolving creativity—the forest dweller seeks to grow in new ways.

There is the need to continue in the world as a dynamic force, while at the same time pulling back from worldly ties and accelerating Self-realization through ego-transcending spiritual practices.

I asked my teacher, Swami Kriyananda, about life in the high civilizations of Vedic India. What was different from modern times?

"In modern times nobility and aristocracy depend on wealth, on how much you own, on purely superficial things. In Vedic India, it was different. It was a way of life in which people thought of expanding their sense of gain by including the gain of others, coming finally to the point of forgetting personal gain, of just thinking, 'I live through others; I want them to be happy and fulfilled.' These are the thought processes of a truly noble person."

He continued. "As noble souls develop, they begin to realize that there is no 'I' and that we are all part of a greater reality that is spiritual. We come to understand that God is serving God. At this point the noble person becomes a true Brahmin; a true Brahmin is a priest, but not a priest in the conventional manner of someone who performs rituals and lectures well. As a true Brahmin you have the attitude that it is God working through you, and that it is for God that you are working."

Everything we do, if done with deep love, service to others, appreciation, and devotion, has the power to transform us, and can in turn help uplift others and the planet.

A friend of mine, a talented artist, offered a beautiful gift before her untimely death. She was Russian and together with her sisters had moved to the United States, escaping the confines of a communist society that disavowed reading books like *Autobiography of a Yogi*. One of the gifts she offered was a larger-than-life-size statue of Shiva that she had sculpted from cement and situated at the entrance to the Kailash housing cluster at Ananda Village.

I remember watching her create the statue, lovingly pouring her energy into it. The Shiva sits in the lotus pose with one hand extended in blessing, his eyes closed in meditation. Through the years after the sculptor's death I have watched a transformation occurring around this auspicious statue. People have painted the statue, added colorful stones at the base, hung prayer flags, planted bulbs, and added to it in various ways. To this day it is a source of uplifting energy for all.

Another friend has taken the concept of service to a new level. Years ago I interviewed him for my book *Reflections on Living: 30 Years in a Spiritual Community*. He had been in the monastery, had run the Apprentice Village at Ananda, had taught college-level English, and was at one time a Kriya Minister. Feeling the pain in the forest after it had burned in the fire of 1976, he felt drawn to work to heal the damaged wooded land of Ananda. He didn't do this by pulling weeds or creating a garden. He used heavy equipment to clear away the overgrowth of brush that followed the fire, an overgrowth that had left Ananda Village even more vulnerable to wild fires. The land that he has been clearing and caring for has become a healthier forest, more fire-safe and more visually pleasing and park-like.

The Forest Dweller stage is an ideal time to explore the lives of saints. When the Indian holy woman Mata Amritanandamayi, known affectionately as Amma, first came to the United States in the late eighties, she held darshan at a small home in the South San Francisco Bay Area. A few of us from the Ananda ashram attended. Though there was some musical kirtan, she kept silence most of the evening, before performing the Devi Bhava, a ceremony in which she becomes the Divine Mother, complete with regalia costume and headdresses. She also performed Krishna Bhava that night, changing costumes and becoming the embodiment of Krishna. Her early life was filled with love for Krishna, and she often danced by herself in bliss as she became the great god.

The Forest Dweller is also the stage of the mentor, the compassionate leader. Outwardly, the mentor is the skillful teacher who is able to lead, inspire, and bestow knowledge on their followers. Younger people often have mentors that teach skills and model confidence. To be a mentor one does not necessarily need to speak or teach. A mentor can be a muni, teaching in silence. Many great yogis have been non-speaking saints, using only their eyes, their actions, and their consciousness to convey knowledge.

My teacher would sometimes comment on how someone had changed, how that person's eyes had become softer, more beautiful, and indicative of inner soul qualities. Once, on the verge of tears, he remarked to a large group of us how, through the years, the eyes of devotees change, showing less ego and more spirit. I intuitively felt he was referring to an older gentleman who was in the room with us at the time. He had for years battled many difficulties. Yet the man's eyes were the masterpiece of his soul: compassionate, loving, and completely gentle.

In *Autobiography of a Yogi*, the deathless saint Babaji gives us a hint of the Forest Dweller stage. He had asked Sri Yukteswar to write a book demonstrating the underlying unity of the scriptures of East and West. One day, when Yukteswar had finished writing the book, he again met Babaji, sitting under a banyan tree. When Yukteswar invited Babaji to honor his house with a visit, Babaji declined, replying, "We are people who like the shelter of trees; this spot is quite comfortable."*

What does it mean to be a Forest Dweller, or one who prefers the company of trees?

Picking up the conch and holding it to the ear, one hears the humming of the ocean. The Vedas say this sound is the natural vibrating cosmic energy of OM—magnified by the conch.

---

* Paramhansa Yogananda, *Autobiography of a Yogi* (Nevada City, California: Crystal Clarity Publishers, 2005), 329.

CHAPTER 19

Wands of the Devas

WHILE LIVING AND WORKING in New Zealand for a year, our son had graduated from college and was exploring the world. He met a Kiwi medicine woman who told him an interesting story. From the time she was a young girl, she'd had a connection with plants that allowed her to communicate with them. When she was in university studying medicine, the teacher asked her to identify a particular medicinal plant. Instead of telling the teacher only the name of the plant, she continued to describe all the healing properties of the plant, what it could be used for and how it could be harvested. The teacher was stunned. All she had asked for was the plant's name.

The teacher responded, "How did you know all these things about this plant?" The girl answered, "The plant told me." Everyone in the class was silent. She looked at the other students for confirmation, thinking that everyone did this. "You know how they talk to you." There were blank stares. It was then that she knew she had an unusual gift for plant communication.

Many years ago, while traveling with friends in Canada, Nakula and I had a remarkable experience as well. We drove north of Seattle to the town of Anacortes to wait for a car ferry that would take us through the San Juan Islands to Vancouver Island, British Columbia. As our ferry moved west towards Vancouver Island, our eastward view of Mount Baker began to fall behind us, a quickly diminishing view of a peak of snow-covered grandeur.

Along the way, we stopped at Orcas Island in the San Juan Islands. The islands here were very green, like floating shrubberies. The ferry unloaded a few cars, then moved on.

A short vacation in nature with new scenery was stimulating. Vancouver Island was where, as a young girl, I had seen my first bald eagle. Throughout this area we always saw orca whales, swimming and diving alongside boats. They used to be everywhere. Now, we were ready with binoculars in one of their primary habitats. Not once did we see a resident orca. After touring through the islands for several hours, we landed at Sidney and drove down island to Victoria, an elegant fragment of London culture set amidst the southern coastline of the wild Canadian west. We were able to secure a room with plenty of space to meditate and a small kitchen to cook our own food.

We walked throughout Victoria visiting parks with totem poles, Anne Hathaway's Cottage (a replica of William Shakespeare's home), and Madam Tussauds Wax Museum. Walking and being in motion gave our young son a way to channel his energy. Children with lots of energy need activities. We visited the Miniature World theme park, hiked out to the ocean, and one evening took a horse-drawn carriage ride through the streets of Victoria with our traveling companions and Rama, our son.

The next day we ventured northeast of Victoria. It was August and we'd been walking through the more than fifty-five acres of the Butchart Gardens, north of Victoria, British Columbia. Here, more than nine hundred varieties of flowers and plants are graciously set amongst curved walkways, totem poles, rose gardens, a Japanese garden, Italian gardens, and even a children's garden. Though our traveling companions had no children of their own, they were not afraid to hang out with our seven-year-old son or answer his straightforward questions, questions such as "Why do you take those vitamins?" Our friend's answer: "These are for old people. We take them because we're old." At one point in our tour of the gardens, Rama disappeared with the couple. We decided to climb stairs along Cliffside Gardens to a high spot with an overlook. Both of us stopped and were silent for several minutes. We leaned over the rail and I noticed that something was happening. Below us were the Sunken Gardens.

Rising from the gardens were thousands, perhaps millions, of what looked like ethereal spots of colored lights swimming around the flower beds below us. Some of these lights were radiating colors while others were levitating and falling through the atmosphere. We both commented on the scene. We felt as if we were inside a surrealistic painting, but with the light strokes infinitely more minute and fine-hued. No, I have never done acid. I rubbed my eyes just to make sure and the scene continued to expand. The veils had parted and we were being shown something. Keeping silence, as if our very movement might extinguish the experience, we went down the hill into the gardens.

Wanting to get nearer to the light beings, we walked slowly. They were all around us; up close their colors seemed very intense. In a harmonious dance, the angelic beings were feeding off the vibrations of the flowers and giving energy to the flowers. We sat on a bench and watched. My previous experience with gardens had been fairly mundane. The devas (nature spirits) lived here in abundance, busily creating an astral heaven for all to enjoy. By helping human beings in the co-creation of gardens, these entities hasten their own evolution. There is an exchange that happens when human beings interact with beautiful gardens. We give the plants and flowers our love and appreciation. We marvel at their beauty and their ability to make us smile.

Astral entities are present throughout the universe, but are especially drawn to places of beauty, places where human love for gardens, flowers, and plants is strongest. I remember my teacher telling us that nature spirits thrive on love—that if they feel unloved and ignored, they withdraw in much the same way people do when their expressions of good will are misunderstood or not reciprocated.

All the visitors came here to soak up the energy, giving in return their love and appreciation to the flowers. "Human beings, even if unenlightened, express the Infinite Consciousness more fully than do the lower animals," my teacher has said. "Having achieved some measure of self-awareness, human beings have a duty to help uplift creatures of lower levels of evolution. Kindness to animals helps them in their spiritual unfoldment, and helps us, too, for it increases our attunement to the Source of all love."

One activity my teacher told me was ideal for those in the third and fourth stages of yoga was gardening. He recommended that each person have a garden plot, or work with others in larger gardens on a regular basis. Beyond their practical value to a self-sustaining community, Kriyananda's vision saw the gardens as a manifestation of the divine feminine aspects of creation. Consciously creating and caring for vegetable and other gardens was one way our planet could bring the feminine aspect more solidly into creation.

In the mid-eighties I went to a lecture by Swami Satchidananda of Yogaville, held at the Cow Palace in San Francisco. During his talk he emphasized the importance of gardening, working with our hands, and our intentions with the earth. He encouraged us all to treat the vegetable seeds with reverence, to pray for them before, during, and after we planted our gardens. He talked about communing with our gardens and our plants. He said that when we picked our fruit or vegetables, to consciously thank the tree or plant that had sacrificed its bounty for our health.

Our afternoon at the Sunken Gardens in Canada marked the beginning of an endeavor our family would come to find immensely enjoyable—the creation and care of gardens.

Gardening is not new to Ananda Village. Ananta, one of the head gardeners for many years, once talked to me about yoga and gardening in the early days of the community: "We met promptly at 7:30 for our garden meetings; 7:31 was late. We had five acres and a four-person staff. There were forty different crops of vegetables and berries, and sixty different types of herbs and flowers; we grew about six tons of food each year. The soil was horrible, and it was not the best climate for a garden, so it was a place that we could put the teachings of yoga to work against seemingly insurmountable odds. Gardening takes an enormous amount of self-discipline and years of hard work. Eventually, the garden's organic material was increased and its production was more in line with that of a normal garden. The garden was a huge effort, and many apprentices couldn't stay with it. We kept expanding the garden, then added the dairy. Working at the dairy was hard as well: hand-milking the cows, shoveling manure, and pitch-forking hay bales by hand. We were basically using the farming methods of the 1800s in the 1970s. All of this hard work was analogous to the amount of effort required for the spiritual path. The garden was a great environment to learn about obstacles, determination, humility, and effort.

"We had to learn *nishkam karma*—to not be attached to the fruits of our labors. Since I was also living in the monastery, I had to truly put this into practice; giving everything to God and not owning anything separate from God. When you serve in the garden, you're not doing it for profit or for the produce, you're doing it for the ideal of being in harmony with organic gardening and to provide wholesome organic produce for the community.

"Yogananda had the ideal that families and community would set the tone for this age. Communities would be an opportunity for America to solve the isolation of the modern age and to cure the incredible dysfunction between materialism and spirituality. Yogic theory says that our suffering and unhappiness come from our identification with the ego, which blocks our knowledge of ourselves as the soul. We unfortunately identify with our position in the world, how much money we make, our job description, our possessions, and our status in life. By identifying so strongly with these worldly ideals, we limit the soul's level of joy to the level of status we have achieved."

While he was living, Yogananda offered countless ways to lead a more fulfilling life, one of them being what he called "simple living and high thinking": "Take the best advice I can give you," he said. "Gather together, those of you who share high ideals. Pool your resources. Buy land out in the country. A simple life will bring you inner freedom. Harmony with nature will bring you a happiness known to few city dwellers. In the company of other truth seekers you will find it easier to meditate and think of God."*

Yogananda advocated a vegetarian diet, lots of raw vegetables, legumes, grains, fresh fruits rather than candy, and occasional fasting to help cleanse the body. For those unable to quickly shift to vegetarianism, he suggested fish or chicken a few times a week, but no red meat or pork. The great yogis view food as a vehicle for life force and energy, and fresh foods as offering more energy than canned and processed foods. Yogis are encouraged not to consume

---

* Swami Kriyananda, *The New Path* (Nevada City, California: Crystal Clarity Publishers, 2009), 293.

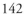

flesh, especially cattle and pigs. These more evolved animals experience immense fear during their captivity and slaughter. This fear radiates throughout their body and through their blood. When we consume their flesh, we are also consuming subtle energies of their fear.

Yogananda also suggested that we work four days at our regular jobs, then spend three days working in the garden. Those familiar with yoga postures and Maha Mudra know that these exercises are a warm-up to the bending, reaching, and weeding needed to maintain a garden. When we were planning to start Ananda University, my teacher gave us several suggestions, one of which was to "grow your own food." Intuitively, he perceived that in today's complicated schemes for education, the most profound secrets for living—the basis for good education—are connected with our earth.

Luther Burbank, the famous botanist to whom Yogananda dedicated his *Autobiography of a Yogi,* was a consummate example of the yogi gardener. Yogananda referred to him as "an American saint." Burbank often talked to his plants to create a vibration of love, letting them know that he would protect them, and that they had nothing to fear. According to Burbank, "The secret of improved plant breeding, apart from scientific knowledge, is love."* Yogananda wrote that "[Burbank's] heart was fathomlessly deep, long acquainted with humility, patience, sacrifice. His little house amidst the roses was austerely simple; he knew the worthlessness of luxury, the joy of few possessions."**

Gardens are havens for positive energy. On the West Coast alone there are the stunning gardens at Lake Shrine in Santa Monica, which Yogananda dedicated in 1950, two years before he left his body. There are the meditation gardens overlooking the Pacific Ocean at Yogananda's Encinitas Hermitage, and the peaceful gardens at Yogananda's original Mt. Washington grounds in Los Angeles. Now, in Ananda Laurelwood, outside Portland, Oregon, residents are creating the Yogananda Gardens. Set high above the Yuba River Canyon with a backdrop of the Tahoe National Forest, Crystal Hermitage, the spiritual heart of the Ananda community, hosts a healing and sacred space created by yogis.

---

* Paramhansa Yogananda, *Autobiography of a Yogi* (Nevada City, California: Crystal Clarity Publishers, 2005), 344.
** Ibid, 348.

The Crystal Hermitage Gardens include a charming chapel inspired by the Porziuncola Church of Saint Francis of Assisi, the Shrine of the Masters, plus several hidden gardens with water features and views. At the far end of the garden, resting on a cliff high above the canyon, is the Moksha Mandir, with its domed blue-tiled roof and golden lotus crown. Inside is a sanctuary for meditation overlooking a thousand-foot drop to the river. Head gardeners have devoted over thirty years to designing and caring for the grounds. As many as fifty volunteers serve, plant, weed, and give tours here. As a service to others, community residents and volunteers spend months preparing for Springtime at Ananda. During April, hundreds of guests visit each day to connect with the vibrant tulips set amidst blossoming cherry trees, wisteria, and other lively blooms. The gardens are open throughout the year, reflecting the beauty of each season.

When we were asked in 2002 to consider living at the remote Ananda Seclusion Retreat in order to start the college, my first thought was "No way!" It was several miles from the main Ananda Village community, farther up in the hills and down a dirt road that seemed never-ending. The road was aptly named Jackass Flats, a remnant of the Gold Rush days when miners used mules to haul their goods. It was riddled with potholes, some large enough to swallow a Volkswagen.

The retreat felt austere. Our thoughts were to make the retreat more accessible energetically, a place where people could meditate and enjoy uplifting grounds, pools, and statues of saints and sages of all religions. We spent quite a bit of time walking the land and tuning in to it.

We soon found that wildlife had more interest in our new garden than did our guests. Wild turkeys invited themselves to dinner. To fend off the deer, we covered the plants with netting. One morning at breakfast in the retreat dining room, a huge buck danced by the window, garden netting flowing from his horns like a wedding veil. The deer "wedding" changed things. Nakula drew plans for a deer fence, garden spaces, trellises, entry gates, a new road, and parking.

We elicited help from Charles Evans, our resident gardener, who had once run a florist shop and art gallery in New York City. For inspiration we took

Charles and Ruth to visit the Mendocino Gardens on the coast of California. Touring the gardens, we discussed possibilities for the Meditation Retreat.

Back at the retreat, we got to work. Tractors were already on site, taking down crumbling old buildings, moving earth and rubble. The demolition left a gaping hole next to the main temple. By reshaping the pit, we created the first landscape feature of the new meditation gardens—the Babaji Pool, a water feature to hold the sacred vibrations of the site—right next to the Babaji Cave. As the months and years went by, the garden grew and filled out. Residents, guests, and students joined in its creation. Charles and Ruth trimmed trees and helped create a canopy that serves as a natural aviary for wild birds, and a playground for squirrels and other forest critters.

One spring I noticed how much taller the blossoming trees had grown. There was a loveliness growing at the retreat. Charles has an intuitive sense for plants and trees, and has become their steward. We added trails and gardens-within-gardens, water features, statuary, and love.

College students created vegetable gardens and together built a solar greenhouse for one of their sustainability classes. We discovered that raking leaves from the pebbled paths is a great form of karma yoga—a tangible and fulfilling chore that, like washing a car, helps the rake clean out personal karma. People come to the retreat for seclusion and for healing. One woman came who had visited only once, twenty years before. She sat on a bench in the garden and wept. I asked her if she was okay, and then listened. She said that although her life was in the city, the one day she had spent in the retreat garden had been the most meaningful experience of her life. "This is my true home," she told me.

When the third and fourth stages of yoga arrive, we can give more time to spiritual practices that go beyond the body. Yet much remains that we can do through the body. The yogi's hands and sensitive fingers have a wand-like ability to transmit energy. We can use them for healing others, for planting, for creating a connection to the Divine. We can learn to send love and healing energy to others. Like the energy that flows out through our meditations, creating and caring for gardens can bring others much joy and peace. The gardener never knows whose spirit a lovingly attended garden may touch.

CHAPTER 20

Wild Things Are

ONE YEAR OUR TRAVEL abroad program went to Cochin, the capital of Kerala, on the far southwest corner of India. As part of our study of World Cultures and Consciousness we visited a Jain temple. The ascetics on the Jain path strictly adhere to ahimsa—non-violence, non-harm to others, including all sentient beings, plants, insects, even bacteria and microorganisms. One might say the Jains are beyond vegan.

Their vegetarian diet is restricted to fruits and vegetables grown above ground. They do not eat root vegetables such as potatoes, onions and carrots, because they are "anathkay": one body containing many lives. When one uproots a vegetable, the entire plant is killed. Honey is not taken because the taking requires violence against bees. They filter their tap water to remove bacteria.

The Jain priest at the temple explained to us that nonviolence is essential to their path—without it one cannot have liberation from reincarnation. Jain monks wear a cloth over their mouths and tied around their heads. This cloth prevents their unwittingly killing tiny insects that might fly in the mouth during breathing. Jains view all life as yoga and seek spiritual development by cultivating the five vows of non-violence, truth, non-stealing, chastity, and non-attachment. Being in the presence of the Jain priest in his temple was uplifting and energizing.

Afterwards, we walked through the ornate temple and outside to the grounds. From the sky high above came a swarm of hundreds, perhaps thousands, of pigeons. They flew into a small area where another Jain monk was feeding them. The mission of Jainism is the same as the mission of nature—to work for the welfare of all, to rise above ignorance in order to obtain perfect bliss and knowledge. Jainism presents a yogic model that highlights the interconnectedness of the vast universe and the belief that nothing is a mistake, not even for a single moment.

As for many yogis growing up in America, nature was my tonic. Becoming one with nature was not so easy. Living at a remote meditation retreat for the past sixteen years has offered countless opportunities to come face to face with wild nature. When I arrived from the Bay Area in the eighties for a Kriya Yoga retreat, I was not prepared for austerity. I had been living in the city and loved it.

After the yoga program I was feeling blissful and confident. I had heard about the trail from the retreat to Bald Mountain, asked for directions, and hiked there. I found the sacred spot and meditated there, even making a circuit of the Indian stone circle. When it was time to return, I couldn't find the trail. I looked for it for nearly an hour, retracing my steps, using my logic to find the elusive path. My mind, realizing I hadn't really told anyone where I was headed, began to play tricks and panic set in. I decided to call on my guru for protection and began a soft bleating of "Om Guru" that quickly turned to a whine, at times a shout, a few tears, and then the knowledge that being a good mile from other human life, I might as well sit down and meditate to conserve my strength, lest it be needed for the cold night ahead.

Finally, I was able to quiet myself, becoming centered enough to offer a sincere prayer. Several minutes later, I stood up and was pulled by an unknown force through the wiry Manzanita underbrush. All along, the trail been only four feet away from me! I had been lost in a maze of dirt ravines and underbrush that looked like a trail but was actually a network of small animal pathways. My lesson was right in front of me, not on a city street, or in a board room filled with powerful executives. Abashed and humbled, I limped back to the retreat.

Many years later, when my husband asked me if I'd like to help him run the Meditation Retreat and start the college we'd been planning for the past year, I remembered wandering alone on the trail to Bald Mountain, and I strongly resisted. At that time the retreat had almost as many hungry bears and mountain lions as human residents.

When I finally overcame my resistance to living in a forest, we moved up to the retreat. By this time I had more inner strength to test myself on the rough trails that surrounded the retreat. Still, I was so careful not to put myself in danger that fear began to sneak into my consciousness. Behind every noise and unseen shadow seemed to lurk forest creatures that all but made me turn and run or even leave the retreat, never to return. Exhausted after several months of living this way, I wanted to change the energy. If I were to maintain my exercise routine—taking long walks outdoors—I needed to make friends with the wilderness and bring it lovingly into my heart.

One day a chant came so strongly into my mind that it became my guide. I took this chant with me on four-mile hikes; when I thought wildlife was near I sang it out loud and strong, sending a message to hidden creatures to spare me and look elsewhere for their dinner. I had read that a woman running by herself near the American River had been attacked and partially eaten by a half-starved mother cougar. Thinking of that woman's death, I chanted even more loudly, affirming my own rightful place in nature: *Oh God beautiful, Oh God beautiful, at thy feet oh I do bow, at thy feet oh I do bow. In the forest thou art green, in the mountain thou art high, in the river thou art restless, in the ocean thou art grave.*

When I first started chanting during my hikes my voice would quaver when I was walking up a steep area so my breath would bounce around with the words—I sounded like a dying animal. I changed my strategy: *To the serviceful thou art service, to the lover thou art love, to the sorrowful thou art sympathy, to the yogi thou art bliss.* I would sing out loud and strong while on level ground, whisper the chant on the gentle uphill slopes, and chant mentally on steep climbs. After several months of walk-and-chant therapy, I began to relax and to feel less fearful.

My next challenge was to involve all the forest creatures with my energy, spreading out so that I embraced the trees, the wildlife, even the insects.

There came a time when I practiced walking in order to approach silently—as the Native Americans did, toe to heel, with the weight resting on the back leg. I took smaller steps to begin with, trying to walk noiselessly, then speeding up to a comfortable pace.

At other times I'd stop and pray for guidance, closing my eyes and feeling the energy deep inside. Watching my breath, practicing calmness, my walks began to be filled with an expanded awareness; sights and sounds arrived in slow motion. I practiced keeping my shoulders back and my heart forward, as though it was the intuitive heart that led me on my walks.

There's really only one direction we are all going on the journey of life, to our own inner self. After many years of living in the forest, I began to notice my heart opening more and more. Inwardly I'd call to the mountain lions as if they were kittens and I was their mother, looking for them. My heart was reaching out. They never appeared to me, but at times I'd see their tracks in the snow or in the wet mud of the trail. With the gradual opening of my heart to the forest I could feel my love spreading to the trees, the sky, even the kitkidizze plants.

I realized how fear can stifle and contract energy. During the third stage of yoga, opening to the physical forest provides a metaphor for confronting all that remains in our subconscious that we haven't faced or released. At the same time, the Forest Dweller seeks the next step on the journey—perhaps the courage to do something new.

There were new creatures to face as well. The bears that lived in the canyons below the retreat were entertaining or frustrating, depending on our human attitudes. If it was a cold winter, they'd hibernate; we wouldn't see them until the late spring. The summer heat brought gardens, fruit trees, and birdseed, all foods they relished. Once we had completed the fence around the three-acre botanical garden, the bears discovered how to open the entry gates, walk right into the garden, haul down the hanging birdseed feeders, give them a good smashing, and eat the contents in return for their efforts.

However destructive they may appear, in the wild they are shy; when they'd see me walking they'd run like a frightened dog. Only once did I see the eight-hundred-pound mother black bear and her cubs, on their way down the hill from a loose compost pile we hadn't fenced off. I was in our car, our eleven-year old son in the seat next to me. I rolled down the window and talked to the mother bear, who was about twenty feet away. My son, frozen in the seat next to me screamed, "Mom, what are you doing? Let's get out of here!"

Caught with her paw in the compost jar, the mother bear had a perplexed look. Bears have an acute sense of smell; they are able to detect an animal carcass twenty miles downwind. "What are you doing, mama?" I said to the mother bear. "Are you showing your cubs the compost?" It was a natural thing to do. Soon after, we shifted the compost pile and bear-proofed it so that they wouldn't return. Wild bears only become a nuisance if we leave tempting foods unprotected and accessible. When they are hungry, look out. If left to forage naturally they eat berries, seeds, and dead animals.

Coyote, the trickster, is far less predictable. We'd hear them barking in the early mornings; when they ventured near the retreat, we'd keep our cat inside. While living in the village, I'd see coyotes work in packs of three to surround and chase prey. They once tried to get two fawns and a doe resting a few feet from our house.

Three coyotes made their way up the hill from St. Francis Pond towards our house. Because at the time our cat was younger and less cautious, I put him inside and went out to dissuade them. While I talked to them their ears stood erect. They stopped and stared at me as if to say, "Look lady, that's my next meal, so if not now, then maybe tomorrow, we don't care." I stood my ground, guarding the fawns. The coyotes eventually tired of listening to me and headed back down the hill. I waited until they were well away, secure in my delusion that I'd somehow saved the entire animal kingdom from extinction.

Nature produced an autumn of extraordinary beauty the year the tiny creatures came into our home. An army of praying mantises arrived to relieve us of paper wasps that had been gathering above our deck. Tree frogs bounced in and out of our house with complete abandon. As fall grew colder, the praying mantises flew into our bedroom when the screen door opened even for a few minutes. Praying mantises live less than a year. When the cold came, they'd squeeze into warm spots. True to form, they found their way to our meditation room and spent their final days sitting on a salt lamp arranged securely on our altar. It was a late October evening when we found two large mantises, one on each of our bedside tables, guarding us, perhaps thanking us for not being afraid.

As the rain and snow came, an alligator lizard also wanted in. I told him he could stay if he took care of the ants and other small bugs. In the spring I saw him outside on the porch. "I think he has a way of getting inside when he wants to," Nakula commented.

One winter's day I put on my snow boots for a walk out towards Bald Mountain, a thousand feet above the South Yuba River. Walking through two feet of snow—four feet in places—gradually the cold dampness crept past my snow gaiters. Jackrabbit and squirrel tracks crisscrossed the trail in front of me. An occasional deer track skirted the edge. I searched for signs of the elusive mountain lion or the solitary bobcat.

In late fall, snow falls so silently that I can hear the far-off trudging of a freight train, traversing the High Sierra from Donner Pass towards Colfax, I look for tracks. When I spot bobcat prints I know that all is well—we have connected. To the Native Americans, the bobcat is symbolic of seclusion and solitude. Many yogis take seclusion two weeks each year in which they maintain complete silence and pull their energy inward. Some friends take month-long seclusions and others, especially those in the Forest Dweller stage, go alone to a secluded spot for several months. During a long seclusion we have the time to reflect on our life's dharma—how are we progressing with the goals we set for ourselves before we incarnated?

For several years, I watched the lone bobcat that lived near the retreat. Once, I mistook it for a large domestic cat; on closer examination I saw that it was much taller. The bobcat liked to trot the dirt roads that skirted the retreat. After years of watching me warily, it finally allowed me to follow it. On an early September morning, after finishing my usual morning meditation, I headed down the trail towards Bald Mountain, moving quietly. Fifty feet in front of me, the bobcat loped along, in no hurry at all. I slowed my gait. After I had been following it for a few minutes, the bobcat paused, looked around at me, then continued on.

I spoke silently: *Hello, baby cat, how are you?* Now and then it would stop and look behind to make sure I wasn't getting too close. We both continued on. As it came to a small hill, it let me get closer. At one point I was only twenty feet away. When I was ten feet away it jumped into the underbrush, then stopped, turned, and stared at me. Our eyes met. It was the wildest face I'd ever seen, full of scars and markings from a life in the underbrush. We stared at each other, both in awe. It was the last time I saw it.

"Look at, or imagine, a river flowing constantly. Then visualize your thoughts flowing similarly—not rippling restlessly; not drifting sluggishly; not frozen in fixed opinions like an ice sheet in wintertime. Adapt yourself to circumstances. The more centered you are in your Self, the easier you will find it to change as the needs arise. Affirm silently, 'I adapt like flowing water to new situations and ideas.'"

—Swami Kriyananda, *Living Wisely, Living Well*

CHAPTER 21

Finding God in Nature

FOR THE FOREST DWELLER Stage of Yoga, I wanted to interview a yogi who has spent most of his life writing and teaching about nature awareness. It was under a lush canopy of trees, that I began my talk with Joseph Cornell, founder of Sharing Nature Worldwide, book author, longtime yogi, and meditation instructor. Since 1975 he's been a practitioner of Kriya Yoga. Now, at age sixty-five, his most recent book has just won six awards, including Grand Prize Winner for Non-fiction, Indie Book Awards.

Though sometimes plagued by health challenges, his energy is vibrant and strong. He does not show any signs of letting up.

Joseph explains to me that trees are beings of light and can heal you: "When I was quite ill and had problems breathing, and couldn't meditate deeply using typical yogic practices, I looked also to nature. Even though my lungs were compromised, I found other ways to go beyond the body, ways integral to yoga practice. I tried to be innovative with my spiritual practices.

"Yogananda once said that we can reduce pain by concentrating on creative ideas, so I developed and began practicing Forest Bathing immersion exercises. Previously, before the onset of an autoimmune illness, I had experienced an exalted period of meditation. Since I could no longer easily transcend the body through regular meditation, I practiced absorbing practices like Forest Bathing and creative writing to serve others. I discovered that creative pursuits and engagement with nature helped me to transcend bodily suffering to a remarkable degree. I became more and more joyful during the seven-year period of severe illness."

I asked him about his early life: "I designed my own degree at the college I attended. The title of my degree was 'How to Find God in Nature.' I decided that those professors who taught with joy and love could be in my major. In my earlier life I had spent a lot of time in the wilderness; something was propelling me to share what I knew and had learned.

"I joined a monastery, and at the same time I was traveling to Australia and England to teach from my book *Sharing Nature with Children*. The book had become quite popular. The whole "hug a tree" movement grew out of one of the book's exercises I created. *Sharing Nature with Children* started a worldwide revolution and was adopted by thousands of nature educators. Because of this book, nature study became more experiential. Japan alone has over ten thousand members of Japan Nature Games, which was part of the Sharing Nature Worldwide organization I started."

Service to others is a constant theme in yoga, and in Joseph's life. When he was young and successful in his work, his spiritual teacher, Swami Kriyananda, asked him to consider another form of service, telling him, "Your work helps a lot of people, but you've come to this ashram to find God."

Joseph shared with me his response to his teacher's guidance: "As we go deeper into the study of yoga, we realize that likes and dislikes are delusions that take us out of our inward focus. It was good for me not to identify with my career so strongly, perhaps especially now that Sharing Nature and my books were becoming famous around the world. My outer career had to do with teaching nature awareness. In Palo Alto I started teaching meditation, and in doing so I was learning to internalize my energy. I've flown over a million miles and visited thirty countries; my books are in print in twenty-four countries around the world. Yet it's the inner experience times that have empowered my work. There's a meditation technique called the OM technique that I'm very fond of. I try always to stay in the OM vibration, a practice I find draws true friends. I give my whole creative process to OM. All the exercises I've developed and created have come to me through prayer and meditation.

"Now, I'm going into a time of more writing. I'm more housebound. Occasionally I have visitors from other countries or special programs, but more and more I'm going inward. Despite my health challenges, I've had experiences, such as going breathless. Sometimes my wife has had to gently nudge me back!" He laughed, his joy level contagious.

"In a new way I'm leveraging all those years of traveling and forming human friendships and relationships so that now I can work at home, pass the knowledge of Sharing Nature to others—and empower them to pass the knowledge to the next generation. Sharing Nature is a worldwide work that's based on spiritual affinity. A friend once said to me, 'After you're gone, Sharing Nature will be much better, much more popular worldwide.' Nature is the best way to teach children, I believe," he added, and I agreed.

"Why do children learn foreign languages more quickly than adults? Because they don't use the analytical, intellectual part of their brains. If we can get adults to stop analyzing and thinking so much, they will be better learners too. We need to emphasize learning more with the heart and intuition. The purpose of experiential education is to expand our consciousness to unite with everything that is. This is the purpose of yoga, to become one with all that is. My work with nature is to give children ways to absorb ideals so that the soul becomes more refined."

I asked what he thought were the hallmarks of great teachers: "Those who have a growing degree of experience with yoga—union with life—and are cultivating this experience in their lives," he answered. "Any effort people are making towards union with all life will help greatly. Everything they do will come out their actual experience. It is also a good practice to cultivate a personal study of inspiring writings, such as the lives of saints. The ability to share will be determined by one's level of consciousness."

"What was your biggest inspiration to write *Sharing Nature with Children*?" I asked him:

"Nature! I wanted to help people by sharing with them how to have profound experiences through nature. By doing so they will become better people. I feel that refined souls will be naturally sensitive to the four stages of learning I have created—Awakening Enthusiasm, Focusing Attention, Offering Direct Experience and Sharing Inspiration.

"Meister Ekhart says the outcome of contemplation is love. I want people to open their hearts; with their hearts open, they'll naturally want to do things on their own," he said with a smile. "People of rigid opinions go around the world annoying others. If you teach with a sense of freedom, you'll have more joy, and so will your students.

"So often people have a cause they're trying to promote. Personal agendas stifle freedom—they obstruct the awakening of world peace. There's wisdom in not allowing ourselves to be hypnotized by a particular cause. When I was ill I'd work on my book fourteen to eighteen hours at a time. Even though I felt terrible, grace surrounded me. I worked with a sense of freedom that I wasn't the doer. It was this attitude of inner freedom that got me through the tough periods. If I was burdened by a cause, or with the sense that I was the doer, I'd be working without the Divine. We need to work with a sense of joy and freedom. The secret of Gandhi's service was his freedom and his love for God. When you can do this, you come to a place of universal peace in your own being."

I asked him what he would like to be doing when he reaches the stage of the Sannyasi.

"When I'm seventy-five I'd like to simply follow the joy I feel in God—whether in writing or in creating, or in deep meditation. Sometimes we still have work we need to do to work out our karma. The last four years I've been very inward here—I do occasionally see others from around the world, but I'm becoming more and more internalized.

"In Greece there's a special place called Mount Athos. A very saintly monk lived there in a cave—one cave he lived in and one cave he meditated in. Mount Athos is very restricted: Only seven foreigners per day are allowed there. This saintly monk had a cell phone, and with the cell phone would talk to his spiritual children around the world! He'd be in his cave, then step out to talk with people via cell phone. When he was finished, he'd step back in the cave and go deep again.

"If I had the opportunity to go deep, I'd take it. The value of going deep in ourselves is that we can then help others so much more profoundly. Before I took my Nayaswami vows I had an interesting experience: I was meditating and a great upliftment came. I felt my whole being flowing into the spiritual eye. Everyone I had ever known was flowing into the spiritual eye; they were going with me. So how do we really help others? The more we are in touch with ourselves, the more true help can flow through us to others.

"Swami Kriyananda gave as the secret to creativity raising the energy in the spine—his own expanding creativity was never obstructed by writer's block. In Patanjali's Yoga Sutras we read, 'We don't have to infer anymore, we just know.'"

As he is one of the leaders of a monastic order, I asked Joseph what counsel he offers monastic householders. He paused and reflected. "Meditate regularly to keep your aura strong. Don't be too hard on yourself—you've got to bring duality to rest. It's something you don't achieve overnight. Use your discrimination, know that it's only in God that you'll find lasting joy. Win gracefully the small battles and enjoy the companionship of your partner."

I asked how he offers help for the young monastics who are single.

"For monastics, if they are to continue in their vocation—they need to be aware of what can distract them from or counteract their intentions. It's important for younger renunciates especially to be in a supportive environment. Don't squander your life forces on outward activities. For monastics, the practice of brahmacharya is to learn to keep the energy centered in the spine. Centered energy is much more magnetic than scattered energy. When you're centered in the spine, outer events will adjust to inner realities. Brahmacharya is not sexual suppression; it means not going out of your own center. A swami is master of himself. It's a gradual process. If young monastics find it difficult to be in silence, they can practice being 'in quiet.'"

Joseph has been married for thirty-two years. I inquired what it's like being married householder monastics.

"We live together as serious devotees. We understand that by putting God first in the relationship, everything else will flourish. Meditate together, support each other, make decisions together that will support an interior life, so that neither of you get caught up in the material demands of the world. At the same time, don't push away those aspects of the material world necessary for you both to carry out your individual dharmas.

"Married renunciates live together like two brother monks or sister nuns. They enjoy constant spiritual *satsang* [fellowship] with someone each has a deep rapport or attunement with." After reflection, he offered a deeper explanation: "Everything we ever want in a marriage comes to full expression when we're both supporting our inner lives." I looked around at the peaceful scene on his simple porch. "Devotees begin to see that godly behavior is better," he concluded.

Joseph explained how he finds inspiration for his books and writing: "I walk out into nature. Sometimes I meditate in that chair near the statue of Lahiri Mahasaya." He pointed to a statue near his small cabin. "I have a creativity area, a place where I can gaze into nature. The nature here is natural," he said. "We don't have bird feeders because the birds then become all rajasic and begin competing with one another. We just want nature to be, and have them come as they come naturally." Then he smiled, "Where the birds are, the angels are."

Over the years, I've experienced Joseph's innocence and joy when he has presented nature awareness programs, imitating birds and animals with child-like abandonment. When he said goodbye to me that day, I half expected him to give a bird call or wiggle his nose like a chipmunk. I looked sideways as I left. With a smile he was gone.

∽

Joseph Cornell, also known as Nayaswami Bharat, is director of the Nayaswami Order, a nondenominational Swami Order.

Nayaswami Vow of Complete Renunciation

From now on, I embrace as the only purpose of my life
the search for God.

I will never take a partner, or, if I am married, I will look
upon my partner as belonging only to Thee, Lord. In any
case, I am complete in myself, and in myself
will merge all the opposites of duality.

I no longer exist as a separate entity, but offer my life
unreservedly into Thy great Ocean of Awareness.

I accept nothing as mine, no one as mine, no talent, no
success, no achievements as my own,
but everything as Thine alone.

I will feel that not only the fruit of my labor, but the labor
itself, is only Thine. Act through me always,
Lord, to accomplish Thy design.

I am free in Thy joy, and will rejoice forever
in Thy blissful presence.

Help me in my efforts to achieve perfection in this, my
holy vow. For I have no goal in life but to know Thee, and
to serve as Thy channel of blessing to all mankind.[*]

---

[*] Swami Kriyananda, *A Renunciate Order for the New Age* (Nevada City, California: Crystal
Clarity Publishers, 2010), 113.

CHAPTER 22

*"I believe that for many people, seventy is the new fifty.
It certainly feels that way to me."*

—Craig Marshall

Brother Craig

I FIRST MET CRAIG MARSHALL many years ago, just before attending the Conference on Precession and Ancient Knowledge (CPAK).

Several of us were taking an early morning hike before the conference started. I was keeping silence, gazing out at the desert and the sky. Abruptly I heard a resounding voice right behind me say: "I think Yogananda is far more than most of us realize." When I turned around, there stood a pleasant-looking gentleman. I nodded in agreement and answered, "Yes, I believe you." Though we exchanged few words, I felt an unspoken kinship in his presence.

Because CPAK focuses on ancient knowledge and research into the vast yuga cycles of time, we always took our college faculty and students. Although the yugas and other ancient knowledge are not discussed in most colleges, in our college we considered understanding where we have been and where we are going a fascinating and mind-expanding experience.

Students in our college have often told me being at this conference and later being able to study and discuss the yuga cycles was one of the highlights of their education.

For the past several years Craig has served as the moderator for CPAK. I had heard he had been a monk with Self-Realization Fellowship (SRF) for thirty-five years before leaving the monastery. I wanted to know more about him, his life as a yogi, and what he did for a living in Los Angeles, California, the city Yogananda referred to as "the Benares of the West."

The High Civilization of Egypt

WHEN I BEGAN OUR interview, Craig was in his car somewhere on the Los Angeles freeway driving to an appointment. We talked on the phone, and I typed into my laptop. In addition to discussing ancient civilizations, Craig shared some stories from his life:

"I used to work in Egypt in my twenties as a photographer. I was attached to a number of archaeological expeditions through journalism, so I got exposed to Eastern teachings then. I remember one time seeing a stone from New Kingdom Egypt (1500 BC). There were inscriptions on the stone, which included the ancient Egyptian hieroglyph for 'breath,' which was ROUA. The inscription said something like, 'When breath is turned back on itself, it becomes light,' and then, 'When ROUA is inverted it becomes AUOR,' (the Egyptian root of the Greek word Auroa), meaning 'light.' The key here is the statement 'When the breath is turned back on itself, it turns into light.' The ancient Egyptians captured many truths in their language. For instance, the ancient word for Egypt was Khemet, which when later arabicized as 'Al Khmet' became the root of the Greek word 'alchemy,' which means transformation." Craig found it inspiring that the name "Egypt" actually means "transformation."

"What's interesting about the Egyptian lifestyle is that all that's left are tombs and temples—all the temples on the east bank and all the tombs on the west bank of the Nile River. In earliest times, Egyptian writing was primitive; and then a magnificent and complete language, the hieroglyphs, burst onto the scene. It's always been a mystery how this came to be. In olden times, Osiris was considered lord of the underworld, and the main Egyptian deity, and his nickname was 'Wenefer' which means 'the Westerner,' perhaps referring to Atlantis. Who knows?

"The Egyptians were aware of the cyclical nature of all things: of birth, death, and reincarnation. Throughout Egyptian temples you see the symbol of the sun, represented by the scarab beetle, which are seen in masses, all walking towards the sun at sunrise. Thus, to this day, the scarab beetle symbolizes rebirth. The clothes and jewelry the Egyptians wore were not designed as fashion pieces. Everything was astrologically based, all symbolic, all related to the elements of creation. The ancients lived their lives connected to spirit. And, even though pharaonic times were in a descending time period (according to the yuga theory), in all periods there are saints, sages, and masters."

I asked Craig his perspective on Egypt, on the passage of time and consciousness.

He replied, "What does it mean to be higher or lower? It all has to do with consciousness. When we're scared or restless, we're part of the problem, not the solution. I felt a real spiritual magnetic call to Egypt. Part of the peace of Egypt is the desert itself. The peace there is incomparable, and the timeless Egyptian civilization has left behind in its symbols and architecture a feeling of depth and divinity. They understood something about integration that we have forgotten.

"The Egyptians, like most ancient cultures, believed in oneness rather than duality. The Egyptians worshipped both Horus and Set, even though Set was the so-called 'evil' one who killed his brother Horus. The Egyptians recognized that contrasting elements, both good and bad, are necessary for the drama we call life; they didn't judge those elements as good or bad, but understood them in the context of a much greater, more expansive reality.

"I think Egyptian culture was unique because it was a crossroads culture. It was the caravanserai on the trade route between India and Europe. Jesus was in Egypt at least three times—when he was a baby escaping the Roman persecution spoken of in the Bible. It is also reported that he was there as a teenager, en route to India; and again on his return to the West, after the 'lost' years of his life. He was ten when he left his home and only came back when he was about thirty.

"The Egyptians understood that the word 'divinity' comes from the root 'division'—they understood that we as individuals are hybrids—we have a higher and a lower self. When we focus on our higher selves, we can be conscious, inspired, and intuitive. When we focus on our lower selves, we can be fearful, get stuck, and resist. The question is not whether we're higher or lower, but where we are at that moment. I think it's important to recognize that we are at a certain point in the cycles of yugas, but it's also important to remember that everything—even time itself—is a dream. As we read in the Indian scriptures, 'Seldom does even a sage realize that the kingdom of heaven is obtainable instantaneously.' We don't need to wait for it. We just need to wake up from the hypnosis of delusion.

"Because the saints, like all of us, can be inspired or uninspired, depending on whether they are focusing on their higher or lower selves at any given time, we can identify with them. It is an illusion to judge anyone as either a 'saint' or a 'sinner.' All of us are both, depending on where our consciousness is at any given moment. Sri Yukteswar once said, 'Forget the past. The vanished lives of all men are dark with many shames. Human conduct is ever unreliable until man is anchored in the Divine.' We can relate to this truth and have hope."

Before he became a monk in Self-Realization Fellowship, Yogananda's organization in Los Angeles, Craig worked as a waiter in the India Café, a restaurant connected with SRF's Hollywood Temple. It was during this time, while learning about yoga and Yogananda's teachings, that he had, during meditation, the vision that inspired him to become a monastic.

For thirty-five years, until 2005, Craig served as a monk with SRF. He was one of SRF's more well-known and popular speakers. You can still view him on YouTube videos, wearing his orange swami robes and talking eloquently about the yogic lifestyle.

I asked Craig what it was like to live for thirty-five years in the monastery, then leave.

"When I was a monk someone asked me why I had become a monk. At the age of twenty-three I was very confused about my direction and getting anxious about the impending decisions I needed to make about job, family, and related commitments. I was clueless and felt I didn't have the depth of understanding and clarity to make such life decisions. Yogananda spoke at length about the importance of environment. The monastery seemed a healthy and supportive environment to help me go deeper."

Yuga Cycles of Time

ALONG THE WAY, SOMETHING must have changed for you. What was it? "I introspected that I had grown up and progressed beyond my youthful understanding of myself. It's the same thing with the yuga cycles of time—this is the core message they bring: that the earth goes through four stages, from a lower level of realization to higher levels.

"The SRF monastics are cloistered; it became clear to me that it was my time to be in the wide, wide world. I still go to services at Lake Shrine, to Convocation; I go to the all-day meditation at Christmas; I have my own private daily practices; and I keep in touch with SRF monks, because they're lifelong friends. In most ways, I feel that I'm more of a 'monk' than ever!"

How would you characterize heroes throughout time?

"The saints, the masters, the geniuses, and the heroes are not part of time because they are not conditioned by their environment. Instead, they are able to step out from their cultured environment and step into their dharma, their life purpose, and their vision. At this point, they begin to influence the world rather than to be affected by it."

Who are your heroes?

"Well, of course, Yogananda. If you look at his life, he was radical, a free-thinker and an inspired visionary from the earliest years of his life. Building a teaching around a guru like that is challenging on many levels. The true guru treats every individual uniquely. Organizations can help people understand the big picture, but as we mature, specific guidance comes increasingly from within, rather than from outside ourselves.

"Because we are all essentially hybrids, with higher and lower selves, integrating these selves without judging and punishing ourselves is a big challenge. Part of the challenge is that when Westerners practice Eastern techniques, there is a little bit of 'wobble in the force.' We're living in a new age: We don't need an Old Testament message, but rather a less judgmental

'Newer Testament.' I remember about twenty-five years ago, I began to strip certain words from my vocabulary."

What are those words and why did you remove them?

"Right, wrong, good and bad—because those terms are dualistic, and polarize conversations, and are the opposite of integration, which yoga encourages. As a young person, I was very judgmental, and I never knew why. My parents weren't that way. For some reason, I had a double dose of it; it was very painful. That kind of dualistic thinking forced me to take it on as a project. Now, praise be, I have become a very, very open person.

"Recently, one of my personal consulting clients asked me a really good question. The question was, 'What is the one quality that your clients could have that would allow them to get the most out of their work with you as a consultant?' I told that person, 'I'm very clear on the answer—it's openness.' And he said, 'How do you define openness?' And I replied, 'It's the capacity to *un*learn. Unlearning is a core skill in transition times like those we are experiencing now on this planet."

Do you give advice?

"I really believe that advice is abuse—because it presupposes that people don't have the answers within themselves. The best way to teach is through listening, questioning, and storytelling. It is said that the most beautiful words in any language are 'Once upon a time . . .' The reason is that our minds are hard-wired to learn from stories. The listener takes out of the story what they are ready to hear. So let me tell you a story. I was a swami and a minister for twenty-five years and I gave a lot of talks, sometimes to as many as seven thousand people. I often gave seven services a month, in places all over the world. Thousands of people came up to me afterwards and told me what a great service it was. So I asked each person, 'Really, what was so great about it?' And never once did someone tell me something that I had said in my talk. Instead they told me something that they were inspired about, which was in response to something I had said. So I thought to myself, 'Cool—I'm doing my job!' My job is to motivate and inspire, and empower individuals to connect with their own inner realization. That's why Yogananda called his organization Self-Realization Fellowship instead of God-Realization Fellowship!

"My job is not to reform the world. I know that not everyone would agree with this attitude. As I see it, there are two primary worldviews—one is that the world is fragile and is in a real muddle, and needs fixing rather quickly. The other worldview holds that everything in the world is perfect always—because the world is meant to be a mirror of our collective consciousness and everything we're thinking and feeling. Thus, only when we change ourselves will the world be different."

What are you doing to earn a living?

"These days I'm doing more public speaking, workshops, and personal coaching. People ask me how do I help young people. My answer is, 'When we're young, we're driven by their willpower and intelligence.' I sometimes say to young people, 'Go! Do your own thing, and let's talk in twenty years.'

Life Begins at Sixty-Two

"THE CHINESE HAVE A saying that your second life begins at sixty-two. Until then, we're much more a part of the problem than the solution. Life can be divided into stages, like a Broadway play, with each act having an archetypal purpose. The first act is the exposition of the characters and the situation. With the second act confusion sets in; resolution and climax don't come until the last act. I guess that's the way it's supposed to be. We want to get our money's worth out of this life! All stages have their riches and beauty. But it's really difficult to be calm and intuitive when we're young, because we're being driven by what's going on in the moment and so respond superficially to our environment.

"Recently, I was giving a lecture in Las Vegas to five hundred honor students from beauty colleges throughout the country. Besides beauty, their profession focuses on communication and helping people develop a positive sense of self. I asked these young people how many considered themselves people pleasers? Seventy percent of the hands went up. We're conditioned to please people. The problem comes when we don't outgrow this stage. We need to start thinking and acting from the inside out, instead of simply reacting to what we think others want of us. If we don't, we never develop our own intuition and a healthy sense of our higher selves."

How do you feel American culture has affected us?

"We've grown up in a pop culture since the Second World War. It has been youth-oriented, positive, active, and yet somewhat superficial and materialistic. Eastern cultures, in contrast, are heavily influenced by age, older people, and ancestors. I believe that our Western culture is stepping into a period of maturation, a time when elders will retake their valuable roles as 'wisdom keepers' and offer guidance based on experience that a younger person can't have because of their limited experience."

How can older people do this?

"I would encourage mature people to take stock of what they have learned, and consider how they can help, either as a second career, as a volunteer, or even informally within their families. The idea is to help younger people learn valuable lessons in virtually every area of life. Mature people have understanding, contacts, resources of all kinds—and can serve as mentors, sponsors, or facilitators, thus helping 'fast-track' younger people to achieve success, both personally and professionally.

"I believe that for many people, 'seventy is the new fifty.' It certainly feels that way to me. The key milestone in life is maturity, or becoming more conscious, more in touch with our intuition and higher Self, so that we can see a bigger picture and live in tune with natural law. Maturity leads to greater success in life. There is a wonderful detachment that comes with age, a detachment that allows true yogis to be 'in the world, but not of it.'"

How do you see this concept evolving?

"The meeting of Western and Eastern culture that we're experiencing today will lead to a marvelous integration, the energy and creativity of youth merging with the wisdom and perspective of age. I encourage everyone to align with their personal life purpose. So many spend decades 'working for the man,' performing tasks that are not aligned with their passion and purpose in life. Many women spend decades raising kids: a service that is valuable, but sometimes overdone. Both men and women have marvelous opportunities these days to have 'second lives,' a time to use their strengths and passions to be productive in truly inspiring ways. In yesteryear, people called retirement 'the golden years.' If that means golf, watching TV, and getting old, it doesn't seem very golden.

"Because I've done so much '*un*learning' in the last twenty years of my life, I now feel that I am a much more open, less programmed person. Now I can do *everything* with greater awareness. And the openness and awareness that I'm experiencing actually open up more opportunities for me. I'm meeting new people, serving others in deep and meaningful ways, having more fun, and exploring more places—truly *living* life rather than just *experiencing* and *reacting* to life.

Finding Your Personal Dharma

WHAT ARE THINGS MATURE people can do in their third and fourth stages?

"I would suggest finding a mentor and joining a 'mastermind' group to explore what one truly wants out of life. We all have blind spots, and if we want to go on a heroic journey, we all need to outgrow our cultural programming. The key is focus. Yogananda gave a helpful formula—read for one hour, write for two hours, meditate (or reflect) for three hours. If people learn to write or journal—whatever can lead them into their innermost consciousness—then their intuition will be better able to guide them.

"It's also important to honor the guidance that comes through feeling. Yogananda said that intuition is perfect reason *and* perfect feeling. In the West we're trained to be a thinking, more than a feeling, culture. When we learn to use our feelings as a moment-to-moment guide, we can make decisions that are more in alignment with our primary purpose and dharma."

What is your life purpose?

"I learned my personal life purpose decades ago. I am a person committed to helping others take a stand for what means the most to them. I help others get clarity on their unique life purposes; with that knowledge people light up, become creative, magnetize new friends, and align with their deepest inspirations. It's a very fulfilling way to live. Deepak Chopra has a saying that's appropriate for the third and fourth stages of yoga: 'According to Vedanta, there are only two symptoms of enlightenment, just two indications that a transformation is taking place within you towards a higher consciousness. The first symptom is that you stop worrying. Things don't bother you anymore. You become light-hearted and full of joy. The second symptom is that you encounter more and more meaningful coincidences in your life, more and more synchronicities. And this accelerates to the point where you actually experience the miraculous.'

"I have no plans to retire because I would like my life to be a service until the day I croak. These days I'm traveling all over the world speaking on mindfulness and meditation. I'm being asked by individuals, organizations, corporations to come and talk to them about core subjects. I'm surrounded by inspired and conscious people. I'm truly living my dream."

You were close with George Harrison and Steve Jobs.

"Some people know that I mentored Steve Jobs and that I was close to George Harrison during the last period of his life. These are both fascinating people, and our conversations went into some very deep territory. Steve had different chapters in his life and was very controversial. Yet, he was always spiritual in his core. He called SRF and wanted to put the audio *Autobiography of a Yogi (AY)* on iTunes, which SRF subsequently did. When Steve died, the only book on his personal iPad was the *AY.* He even arranged that all the guests at his funeral would receive copies of *Autobiography of a Yogi.*

"For many years, Steve talked to me about personal things. George Harrison and I had a brotherly relationship. I hold in confidence what both of them said to me. I truly felt that we all learned a lot from each other. I've learned that all people need to follow their own dharmic path and be faithful to their personal life purpose. It is in finding their individual way that I help people find clarity. I remain amazed that we weren't given these core teachings in school."

What are some of the tools you use?

"I have a complete collection of standard mindfulness and meditation techniques—but in a very personalized way. I find out what people are receptive to and excited about, and I build programs that they will practice. Without practice, it's all intellectual and philosophical. I teach people how to trust their intuition, and that both their thoughts and feelings are guidance systems. I encourage them to look for the subtle clues in their lives, clues which are constantly telling them where to go, what to do, everything they need to know."

How about your family?

"Did I tell you about my mom going to a psychic before I was born? My parents were married in 1931, at the height of the Great Depression. They wanted kids but none came along. In 1941 my dad joined the Navy and was gone for four years in the Pacific. My mother moved to California and built airplanes at Lockheed Aircraft. During this time she went to a psychic who told her, 'Your husband will be home from the war in 1945; you'll have a son and he'll be born in September 1946. You're going to live north of LA and have lots of different jobs, but you'll end up in Hollywood and be very well-known.'

"As predicted, I was born in September and my mother became the top children's agent in Hollywood and was well-known. But the psychic story isn't over. In 1970 I became a monk; in that same year my mom read an article in the *Los Angeles Times* about the same psychic she'd seen years before. My parents went to see him. My father was so spooked that he couldn't go in. My mom knocked on the door and said, 'You won't remember me, but back in the day you gave me a reading.' The psychic interrupted her and said, 'He's become a monk, hasn't he?' She said, 'Yes. He has.' And the psychic continued, 'He's no Catholic, because I see him sitting like this,' and he folded his hands to represent me sitting cross-legged. The psychic shook his finger in my mother's face, and ended by saying, 'Don't you dare try to get him out of there, because he has such wonderful men friends that are going to help him more than you could ever understand or imagine.'

"To me, my mom's experience is proof that there is a life plan for all of us. I believe we 'laid it all out' before we came here, then 'drank the cup-of-forgetfulness' in order to become unconscious enough to enjoy the journey of remembrance, to enjoy putting the pieces back together of our cosmic one Self—to *re*member our divine identities."

Do you ever have beyond-the-veil experiences?

"Yogananda talks about 'Whispers from Eternity,' but I would call them 'winks from eternity.' The wise ones learn that the whole thing is irony; to take it seriously is the primal delusion. It's a great joke . . . if we get it. I guess that we're supposed to take life seriously in the beginning in order to experience the necessary contrast that creates the clarity of who we really are and what we really want. And we all want the same three things—love, peace, and joy. But we are all destined to find these three things in our own ways during our own unique journeys. That's why advice isn't helpful. We all need to figure out our own unique path from within. There are certain generic tools such as meditation and the science of yoga, but all people have to develop their own personal practice in the ways that are most meaningful to them. The true masters do not produce disciples; they produce masters. The Great Ones are examples; their main role is to encourage mature disciples to follow their own inner guidance and personal dharma, and achieve Self-realization."

Chapter 23

Yogic Healing

"To me, selfless service to humanity is the most important vow to follow."
—Nischala Joy Devi

NISCHALA JOY DEVI HAS lived the yoga stages to their fullest, but in reverse order. When I first met her she was wearing the orange robes of the Swami Order and was living as a monastic at an ashram founded by Sri Swami Satchidananda, a disciple of Sri Swami Sivananda. She took her initial vows of renunciation in 1975 and her final monastic vows in 1977. At that time she known as Swami Nischalananda.

She is a pioneer and leader in the field of Yoga Therapy, author of many books, serves as a member of the Advisory Council for the International Association of Yoga Therapists, and has been a moving and inspiring international teacher since 1974. She spent over twenty-five years as a monastic disciple with the world-renowned Satchidandaji, receiving his direct guidance and teachings. She has also received the teachings of many great yoga masters in the United States, India, and elsewhere in the world.

Her landmark research in yoga therapy for life-threatening diseases—Lifestyle Heart Trial—also known as Dean Ornish's Program for Reversing Heart Disease, and the award-winning Commonweal Cancer Help Program—culminated in the creation of her Yoga of the Heart certification course for teachers and health professionals.

I wanted to learn about Nischala Joy's spiritual journey. "What was it like being a monastic when you were just a young woman?" I asked her. "It was bliss," she answered. "I felt I was doing exactly what I was supposed to be doing. I loved the sadhana, and I had no relationship desires. I felt I had burned all that out." Twenty years later, things changed dramatically. She met her future husband, Bhaskar, a monk at Yogaville. "We were friends for many years. We each separately realized we were unable to remain at the ashram and in the monastic order," she explained. "The difficult decision we individually had to make led us both to leave the ashram at different times. Not wanting to traverse the greater secular community alone, and since we held a strong longtime friendship, we began our new life with that friendship."

After five years together, the two friends married. They moved from Virginia to California. Once they were settled, Nischala Joy contacted Dr. Dean Ornish, a fellow devotee of Swami Satchidananda, and someone with whom, in 1991, she had collaborated on the first heart study: Lifestyle Heart Trial. In ten hospitals across the United States, Ornish had been starting a new clinical lifestyle trial to reverse coronary artery disease. The actual clinical study, named The Multi Center Lifestyle Heart Trial, used the principles of yoga, meditation, vegetarian diet, and exercise, and was prepared under Satchidananda's guidance.

I wondered how it was for her to leave Yogaville: "How did you feel about the vows you had taken?" I asked her. "You can't renounce renunciation," she answered. "Times have changed since the large monasteries reigned supreme. There are always many positive reasons for living away from the world in a monastic setting, including our desire to touch that spirit within. I hold that same spirit of renunciation in my life, just without the outward signs."

"How do you see your life unfolding now?" I asked. "I see life as a comedy, not as a tragedy!" she laughed.

"Even though the large monastic communities are phasing out, the need for spiritual community or satsang is greater than ever. I believe new models for yoga communities are needed. At Yogaville, we embraced four vows of the Swami Order—Poverty, Celibacy, Obedience, and Selfless Service to Humanity. The first three rules support the last, *Selfless Service to Humanity*," she emphasized. "To me, that one was the most important to follow. There are a lot of people in the Western monastic model who are in pain and confusion," she added. "They think they won't rise as high spiritually if they don't keep the other three vows."

I asked her, based on her life in Yogaville and her teaching experience at Ananda Village and at many yoga centers throughout the world, what she envisioned for yoga communities in the future. "I believe the vision for this time" she answered, "is to create an open, loving community of sincere people coming together to support each other in deepening their spiritual commitment and embracing their inner light. The community must be expansive beyond any narrow beliefs so that it embraces all people. The tolerance must rise to include those whose beliefs may be broader or include practices beyond the established community's beliefs.

"Attitudes in these yoga communities must include an empowerment of the individual, and if there is a charismatic leader, she or he must be benevolent, with insight and unbending compassion. All races, beliefs, and sexual preferences should be welcomed, on the understanding that we are all one. Fifty years ago teachers like Swami Satchidananda and Swami Kriyananda had a different mission than teachers do today. They were great leaders and role models for that time. Now we need a different type of role model. I don't think celibacy is a necessary virtue. During this age monasticism has lost its original intention and has become a mutation. Two hundred years ago a monastery might have had eight hundred people, but now has only three people. At this time the world's focus is more on developing relationships."

I asked her about relationships and yoga. "One of the greatest gifts we can share with another is the gift of love. This can come in many ways, from a glance to the intimate act of making love. From a yogic point of view, the art of making love is not merely a physical act, but rather a deep spiritual practice, holding your beloved as an aspect of the Divine, elevating that person to goddess or god," she explained.

"Engaging in this way, the subtle and physical aspects of relationship intertwine. The bodies mesh, the minds meld, and the spirits soar. Every aspect of our being is nurtured by this sacred act. To add height to the experience, imagine that each partner is practicing Karma Yoga. The practice of *brahmacharya*, which means moderation as a means to know your higher Self, when applied to another person, is Karma Yoga, learning to serve. Act to give pleasure to the other, and act to please without thinking about the outcome for oneself. If the other partner practices with the same intention, then a perfect action has been created. The outcome of such a practice is realizing we have merged our spirit with another's spirit. We are one."

Relationships can be intimate, but they can also be expansive. "For instance, when we met the Dalai Lama at the airport, he left us with this inspiring thought: 'The problem is that there are seven billion people on this earth, and we think of them as others instead of as ourselves. Until this attitude changes, there won't be peace.'"

She continued, "Still, today, in orthodox religions, sex is only seen as the means to procreate. In some traditions a barricade is placed in the bed between the man and woman when the woman is menstruating, with the strict rule that they not even touch each other. We have put an imaginary barricade between people and called it 'spirituality.'"

I asked her if she was referring to the fact that she no longer wears the robes of her monastic vows. "In this age of relationships," she explained, "we need strong people to show that there can be strong relationships. Before, it was always the monks who were the models. These days many people have difficulty with spiritual authority. At the same time, they're looking for role models. Why not show that you can love each other in the world, not only in a monastery?"

Being in the world and working with a variety of students has caused her to rethink the way she teaches: "Wearing your monastic robes as a badge of honor often pushes people away and makes you appear 'more spiritual.' To practice selfless service, you should be with the people on their own level."

I asked about her life before becoming a monastic. She reflected a moment before answering: "I was raised in Philadelphia, in a home with no religion practiced. My father was an atheist and my mother was agnostic. My mother's idea of celebrating Jewish Passover was to buy a box of Matzoh; her idea of celebrating Christianity was to buy hot cross buns at Easter. It was their openness, love, and their gift to me of the right to choose, that encouraged me spiritually."

"Can you share any illuminating experiences you had studying with your teacher?" I asked. "I have a fond memory from some years ago," Nischala Joy answered, "of accompanying my teacher, Sri Swami Satchidananda, one of the twentieth century's great yoga masters, on a walk in the park. I was one of three people walking behind him, and I was enjoying the beauty of the day and the feel of the soft, slightly damp grass under my feet. Realizing that many creatures were living in the earth beneath my feet, I was aware that my actions could be causing harm to them. As I was thinking about this, I noticed that as Swamiji lifted his foot before taking the next step, the grass perked back up. Looking back at the grass I had just stepped on, it was flat. Curious to see if it was the same for my companions, I glanced over at the others, who were also flattening the grass as they walked across it.

"Perplexed, the three of us approached Swamiji. 'Why is it,' we asked, 'that when you walk on the grass it stands back up when you lift your foot, while the grass under our feet stays pressed to the earth?' A sweet, reverent expression came to his face, and he put his hand on his heart. 'I have reverence for the earth and she knows it,' he said. 'When I walk on her I feel I am walking on my mother's bosom.'

"I don't know if I'll ever fully understand what happened that day, but the incident illuminated for me how deeply you can alter your consciousness to love and respect the earth. Even now, as I walk through the park or on the grass, I am conscious that the earth is my Mother."

I asked her about yoga therapy and her role in healing others. She spoke of the koshas, the subtle bodies surrounding the true self: "With the stresses of everyday life, the energetic flow is often hindered. The result is lethargy, anxiety, depression, or even disease. By observing the adjusting images of ourselves, we are able to release old paradigms from the subtle bodies and gain control of our very life force. As these pathways are unlocked, the pent-up energy effortlessly flows and we are able to heal everything, from simple ailments to life-threatening diseases.

"When we practice yoga," she continued, "whether it's asana, pranayama, meditation, mantra, devotion, or Karma Yoga, we are having an impact on one or more of the koshas or subtle bodies. Understanding that the practice of yoga releases blockages in the many layers helps us understand why we sometimes resist—strongly resist—our practices. Those blockages in our body often hide fears and unexpressed emotions. Sure, yoga will make us feel great, but it will also make us *feel*.

"Sometimes unpleasant feelings, thoughts, or bodily sensations arise during or after yoga," she went on. "It helps to have a conceptual model to understand why this can be. This kosha is called the *annamaya kosha*, or the body of food. It governs our physical body, which is made up of muscles and bones, ligaments, tendons, and vital organs. This is the kosha most people are concerned about when they begin a yoga practice. They want increased flexibility; they want to tone up their muscles; they want to learn to relax their bodies; they're looking to gain strength, improve their balance, and find stress relief. The primary way to impact the annamaya kosha is through *asana*, or yoga postures."

"The practice of asana," she further explained, "will also impact the second kosha, *pranamaya kosha*—the energy body. Just as the Chinese have chi, the yogis have prana—or life force. Prana moves throughout the subtle body via channels, or nadis. Some seventy-two thousand to one hundred and fifty thousand apparently; although, who counted them? Nobody knows. When we practice asana and pranayama, we are impacting the pranamaya kosha. Any blockages in those nadis are cleared out, bit by bit. And your improved flow of energy in the subtle body (energy body) can then affect the annamaya kosha (physical body) and also impact any health issues you may be having," she said.

"How do you characterize prana," I asked her. "We are born," she answered, "with a certain amount of prana; it also comes into the body by way of food and water, but also by breath. One of the major benefits of yoga is that we become conscious of our breathing, and—sometimes for the first time as adults—learn to take proper deep breaths. This increase of prana into our system makes us feel literally more alive; it invigorates and empowers the pranamaya kosha.

"Number three on our tour of the koshas," she said, 'is *manomaya kosha*, the mental/emotional body. People usually come to yoga for the physical benefits, and stay because of how yoga affects the manomaya kosha. You feel great after class—mentally clear and emotionally upbeat. That's what keeps you coming back, time after time.

"The manomaya kosha is that aspect of Self which hones our intellectual and emotional needs; it also helps us fulfill our individual desires, including on a practical level: safety, security, obtaining love, and taking care of loved ones.

"If you're experiencing underlying anxiety because you've lost your job and you don't know how you're going to pay rent, your experience is in manomaya kosha. A calming yoga practice like Alternate Nostril Breathing can help alleviate those feelings and thoughts.

"Most of us have a tendency to 'live' in one kosha more than in the others," she continued. "Some people are body-orientated; Westerners tend to be mind-orientated. However, the practice of yoga helps us to balance out our awareness of all the layers of Self and shift us out of being primarily in manomaya kosha. One effect can be that our anxiety lessens. Even though anxiety may still be there, we may feel more grounded in annamaya kosha; we may also rise into the fourth kosha—*vijnanamaya kosha,* the wisdom body."

"How can cultivating wisdom benefit us?" I asked her. "The ascension to the wisdom body," she answered, "gives us a broader perspective on our life experience; we're able to see that we'll get another job, or that we have plenty of resources to call on. Then the anxiety fades. Furthermore," she continued, "cultivating the fourth kosha—vijnanamaya—is an unexpected benefit of yoga for most people. You turn up expecting an exercise class and wanting to touch your toes. But you find yourself connecting to a deeper level of intuition, greater internal wisdom, and a sense of higher knowledge. Granted, deepening into an awareness of vijnanamaya kosha may take more than a class once a week; but if you continue to practice, it will come."

"Is this the kosha," I inquired, "that helps us actually feel yoga, or union?"

"It's at this more subtle level of our Self," Nischala Joy answered, "that we begin to shift from a primary I-ness orientation—'I am a separate being'—to a primary One-ness orientation. We feel, and understand, on a deep level that there is no real difference or separation between you and me. We move beyond feelings and concerns based on survival and security, and into feelings that encompass and include all—such as compassion, love, and joy. Our relationships change and become more fulfilling, and more joyous. Life simply becomes good. We're well along the path of yoga—the journey from ego/mind or small self to Atman or Big Self."

She went on to explain fear and healing: "Delving into the vijnanamaya kosha means shifting consciousness through doing the practices that remove the blockages in the three previous koshas. When we find comfort and harmony in our physical body, we are able to release blockages in our energy body, and can then heal and release fears and emotions from our mental body. As you shift more and more into vijnanamaya kosha, you will watch life open up before you into an expansive landscape where you love everyone. *Truly* love everyone." Laughing, she added, "Now that's a pretty cool benefit of doing a few Sun Salutations every day, huh?"

"Finally," she said, "There's the fifth kosha, the *anandamaya kosha,* or 'the body of bliss.' Exactly as it sounds, this is the realm of bliss. No longer separate, you're bathing in oneness with All That Is. You and the Divine are one and the same. And that's about all I'm going to say about the fifth kosha, because if you're getting there, you don't need me to tell you about it. And if you're not there, I can't tell you about it, because I'm not there either. Yet."

"What usually happens," I asked, "to patients you've worked with?" "As you practice, no matter what style of yoga you're practicing, you're releasing blockages in one or more of these layers of the body. Old memories—both good and bad—may float to the surface of your consciousness. There may be a spontaneous release of emotion in the form of tears or laughter. You may experience jerking of the body when energy releases in strange ways. All these experiences are normal forms of release. All can be part of your yoga therapy experience. The healing that occurs, ultimately—not only healing of body or mind—is knowing that we are all love, and that we are all one."

CHAPTER 24

The Sannyasi—Age 73–120

"There was a time in India when the sannyasis were the true rulers."
—Swami Kriyananda

IN THE FOURTH STAGE of yoga, the conditions for being a yogi exist naturally. The last stage can be the most meaningful time of life. Now yogis have time to further their quest for Self-realization.

Each of the first three stages of yoga traditionally gives a duration of twenty-four years. In the earlier stages time appears more concentrated. We feel impelled to use energy in outward ways, simply to sustain life and in pursuit of worldly goals. The first twenty-four-year stage is characterized by impatience to grow up and actively enter the world. The second, householder stage finds us proving ourselves as mature adults, raising a family, having a career, paying bills, and learning to serve others. The third stage brings us face to face with the reality of the forest dweller; we are finally able to examine our life for its true purpose—to develop our latent spiritual gifts even as we gradually withdraw from the world.

The fourth stage of yoga comes when energy is withdrawing from our physical body at the same time that our consciousness is expanding its horizons. What a juxtaposition! We have more time when we're older and less time when we're younger.

Swami Jnanananda, a sannyasi who spent most of his life in the Himalayas, says that the fourth stage is dedicated to divine knowledge: "The divisions can be described like this: the first is one of *addition*, for a student must acquire knowledge. The second is one of *subtraction*, for a householder supports his family. The third is one of *multiplication* because, having retired from worldly life, one has nothing else to do but acquire inner knowledge. The fourth is one of *division*: that is the time to distribute these inner riches for the enlightenment of others. So really, to enter sannyas means to dwell in God."

It is said that OM is the most sacred mantra to merge into God. When the yogi chants the sacred OM, it leads to perception of the Infinite. OM is the symbol for the Sannyasi.

Carl Jung characterized the fourth stage of life as that of the spirit. In the last stage, Jung says we begin to step back and see ourselves as spirit, realizing that we are much more than the sum of all our possessions and achievements; the ego begins to surrender itself as it prepares to cross the finish line in the race of life.

A friend and lifelong yogi gave this perspective: "I've followed this path very seriously since my early twenties, which now amounts to many decades. I find it interesting to contemplate how the many facets of our souls are revealed to us at different times, so that we can work on them, and ultimately balance them all and become free."

In traditional Vedic lore, the fourth stage of Sannyas occurred when the yogi left home, having no other attachment, wandering as a sadhu and strengthening attachment to God, not to worldly pleasures—renouncing all desires, fears, hopes, duties, and responsibilities. Kriyananda said that the physical landscape of Ancient India was much more conducive to the practice of a wandering sadhu going from one place to another. Now, the physical landscape has changed. Yogis must adapt.

Swami Satchidananda of Integral Yoga defined the word sannyasi as "'perfect abandoning' or 'setting aside.' The one whom we call monk in English, or a sannyasin in Sanskrit, is one who has renounced his or her personal life. He or she lives for the sake of others—eats, drinks, and breathes for the sake of others—renouncing selfishness and serving all. That is the only requirement for a sannyasin. There's nothing else. Sannyasins come forward to renounce everything that would disturb their peace. They come to retain that peace and then to serve others by helping them find that peace.'"

For the stage of Sannyas, Swami Kriyananda of Ananda has given this guidance: "This is also the time to start thinking more about the afterlife. Yoga philosophy teaches that everyone should be trained throughout life, and especially in childhood, that life is a preparation for the final exam of death. Sooner or later, you're going to leave this world. How will you leave it happily? Only if you think in terms of loving people, of being wise and giving, of being kind, of understanding other people's problems and not just thinking in terms of your own survival, can you rise above the chains of self-involvement and the negative qualities that this brings.

"Love can never die. The love we feel for our spouse, another human being, and mankind as a whole is not lost because we shed our human form. In the afterworld we meet our old friends and loved ones. It doesn't mean that partners will always be together—they could be man and wife, mother and daughter, they could be linked through all sorts of relationships. You may also have new associations. Buddha said that the reason we should love everybody is that everyone in the world at one time or another has been close to us.

"What truly uplifts people is the amorphous longing of the soul for liberation and for bliss. We should be trained all through life, and encouraged to think, in terms of death—not in morbid, fearful terms, but as death of the ego, and death of this human body, that will at some time cease to exist as our soul lives on.

"The time of Sannyas is the time to begin thinking, 'Well, I'm not going to be around all that much longer; how will I go? Will I go fettered or free? And if I want to be free, then I have to give up desires. I have to give up thinking about myself. I have to think in terms of pleasing and serving God.' Most people don't think in terms of God; they don't think in these noble terms. But everybody to some extent can be trained to think in terms of preparing for death—and freedom in death rather than regretful bondage. As yogis, we

---

* *Integral Yoga Magazine:* integralyogamagazine.org/monastic-order/, accessed 2/16/18.

know that love never dies. What dies is the body, the outer shell that has been our home.

"In the 1800s, even the great Indian yogi Lahiri Mahasaya didn't encourage people to become sannyasis. He allowed some people to become sannyasis, but he basically felt that Indian society was too poor to support a huge population of renunciates. And so the days of Sannyas were based on a society where people could give food to the sannyasis, so that they could keep body and soul together. It would be a blessing for householders to fulfill this role in today's society. Anything you do for a spiritual motive, or for a spiritual person, is good karma for you. In India they have the tradition of giving feasts for Brahmins—the idea being that these are supposed to be people whose lives are dedicated to God, and by serving them, you're serving God.

"Ancient India proclaims that sannyasis look upon all souls as their own family, not just their immediate blood relatives. There was a time in India when the sannyasis were the true rulers. All the kings and politicians would bow to them, touch their feet. This is because the true sannyasis lived for others only, not for themselves or their limited family."

CHAPTER 25

A 1987 visit to Mother Teresa during her fourth stage of yoga.

Mother Teresa

THE DRIVE THROUGH CALCUTTA's slums to Mother Teresa's Missions of Charity was shocking to my Western mind. It was 1987, and though, while in college, I had witnessed intense poverty in the slums of Haiti, I had never seen anything like this. All along the streets, hundreds of people were living in cardboard boxes or makeshift homes with plastic tarps for their roof. There was nowhere to stand, families were hunched over like animals in cages, protecting themselves from the searing heat. During the monsoons the slums would became much more perilous when rising floodwaters and the lack of sewers would spread malaria and disease. Many of us on this trip were young and had never seen such destitution.

My greatest desire before I became deeply involved with yoga was to meet Mother Teresa of Calcutta. I was raised Christian but not Catholic; even so, I knew of her spiritual greatness. She was a hero at a time when the world needed her example.

Mother Teresa was a Roman Catholic nun born in Albania. Although she first served in Ireland, it was in India that, after many years, she found her life's work. As she was riding a train from Calcutta to Darjeeling, she heard a call within from Jesus. Jesus asked her to help him serve the poorest of the poor. By August 1948, she had started her Missions of Charity, serving the unwanted, the unloved, and the uncared for.

Mother Teresa set an example of mercy and charity for our modern world. She became a legend when she was given the Nobel Prize for Peace in 1979, not only for her work in the slums of Calcutta, but "for work undertaken in the struggle to overcome poverty and distress, which also constitute a threat to peace."

So it came about that my sincere prayer was to be answered. In 1986, Ananda was planning a pilgrimage to India. I shared with the leaders my desire to meet the Great Mother. Although we weren't sure we would be able to see her, a year later we did.

Nothing during our trip to India challenged our eyes like Calcutta.

Upon arrival at Mother Teresa's main outpost, we were told we were early. We waited outside. Across the street a small family squatted on their haunches beneath a makeshift shelter, so cramped for space the family could barely move about, carrying out their domestic duties. A narrow cot, about nine inches off the ground, held a sleeping body that was skeletal and infirm.

As the street scene unfolded, I couldn't help but stare. Calcutta felt like an underground planet, a place my heart was afraid to visit.

Finally our host arrived; it was time to go inside. A nun dressed in a white sari with blue trim greeted our group. Other pilgrims, some Western, some Indian, began to file into a large room with a cement floor and an altar. Two white male priests dressed in similarly pale robes arranged themselves to begin a Mass. The ceremony continued as more and more pilgrims filled the room. The group shuffled up for the Eucharist. We approached individually and the priest placed the consecrated wafer on our tongues. I cringed at the thought of swallowing the tiny wafer symbolic of Christ's body. I was remembering how, in my youth, the bland wafer would stick to the roof of my mouth.

I was standing in the back of the room, still toying with the glutinous blob in my mouth. I began looking around and wondering where Mother Teresa was, sure that she must be up on a pedestal near the altar. She was not to be seen. The room was now very crowded. I turned to my friend Asha to ask where Mother Teresa was. She shrugged her shoulders. Then, next to Asha, who was much shorter than me, I saw a tiny old nun, less than five feet tall. I gasped, motioned with my eyes, and we both looked down. There she stood, her eyes focused on the altar, as if she too were looking for someone.

We tried not to look, yet what does one do after flying halfway around the world in search of those few seconds of electrifying presence? My heart began to beat faster and I tried to calm it. I breathed quietly and offered a silent prayer. I studied her hands with a side-glance, absorbing what I saw like an artist about to paint.

After the service, the head nun motioned to all the pilgrims to follow her. I lingered for a few moments and watched Mother Teresa, not taking my eyes off her. She walked over to a large statue of Christ on the cross, knelt down and stared up at Jesus, her hands in prayer. Christ was looking down at Mother Teresa, his eyes full of compassion. The Great Mother's hands were formed together in prayer at her heart center, and her eyes looked up into those of the Christ, the two in deep silent communion. I stood frozen and stared. I'd never seen or felt such devout energy before. The skin on my arms was beginning to tingle.

The communion between the Great Mother and Christ seemed to go on for several minutes, as if locked in a tight discussion. Mother Teresa appeared tiny, much smaller than I imagined. Her eyes wore a deep sadness of strength and compassion from a lifetime of service to the poor, the dying, those needing love, and her healing touch. She seemed to be telling Christ all her deepest secrets, worries, asking for his strength.

I noticed that her back was badly stooped in a permanent curvature of the spine. She seemed the most unlikely of yogis. Yet here in the slums of Calcutta, this life of devotion had achieved the true yoga: union with her Master, Jesus, in service to Christ in suffering humanity. As I continued to stare at the Mother and the Christ, I began to feel something intangible enter my consciousness.

Soon the Great Mother slipped quickly away, on to her next routine. I followed her out of the room, and, keeping a respectful distance, continued to observe her.

Her voice was quiet, almost unrecognizable, and those she spoke with had to bend close to hear. She whispered with another nun and motioned to the rooms where the sick and dying were being cared for. The sister guided our pilgrimage group to these rooms. Some carried buckets and mops, yet all watched the Great Mother, their eyes wide and staring.

She had the demeanor both of a saint and of an army commander; nothing stood in her way. She was unaware of anything but giving the deepest comfort to those in her care. These were street people, the poorest of the poor. Some were thin, dying, and elderly. Others were young and crippled. There were lepers without limbs, and many had physical abnormalities.

She walked up to a middle-aged man whose legs were so thin he could not walk, his bones bending painfully as he tried to sit up. The simple stick cot lay in contrast to his own frame, who could tell which was the thinner? He looked in need of a bath and had little for clothes. Mother Teresa touched his head and ruffled his hair. She looked into his eyes deeply, gave him a loving smile, and spoke with him in Hindi.

The old man gave Mother Teresa the biggest of smiles and his eyes dove into her own. She spent several minutes talking with him, giving him her love and energy. A few nuns squeezed next to her, and she gave them brief instructions. She was the greatest of mothers; you knew she held no judgment in her heart.

Mother Teresa shuffled to the next cot and I looked closely at her hands. They were large, like a man's hands, strongly formed, with thick wrinkles stained a deep brown by the Bengali sun. They looked like the hands of a farmer; someone who had toiled daily in the earth, separating rocks from potatoes with her hoe. An image came of her lifting a hoe and hitting the dirt clods, dawn to dusk, picking and smoothing.

Years later I saw footage of the mother in war-torn Beirut, visiting a hospital whose panicked staff had been forced to abandon a large group of handicapped and retarded children, leaving them to suffer on their own. They were infested with flies, full of fear, crawling on the floor. The Mother thought nothing of the television reporters trying to chronicle her visit. She turned and looked at the military man in charge and spoke to him as she would to one of her nuns. She told him to go help the other refugees, to care for them, and not spend his time fighting. She wouldn't even look at the film cameras. Her love and focus were elsewhere.

Back at the Missions of Charity, Mother Teresa walked up to a woman with a deformed mass on her shoulder, lying precariously on her side. The tumor had grown so huge it hugged her ear and pushed at her neck and face. The mother knelt on the floor and grabbed the woman's hands and spoke lovingly to her, smiling. Her soft words were sprinkled with a thick accent from her Eastern European roots. The woman with the tumor responded, squeezing the mother's hands. The mother continued to talk to her, smiling, giving love, always giving. She connected deeply with each person. Her focus was completely on their eyes, their well-being, giving them each the love of the Christ.

I studied her face. It was indelicate, sad, filled with ravines of skin crowded on top of each other, containing the suffering of the world. Her eyes moved calmly, as if propelled by some higher force.

She turned to another cot where an old man lay huddled on a grey blanket. He had only one arm, his left severed at the elbow, condemned to a lifetime of street begging. His face was skeletal and his body too weak to move. The mother touched him on the forehead and he looked at her. Then she placed her hand gently on his heart chakra, sending a message into his fragile frame. Keeping her hand on his heart, she knelt down next to him, closed her eyes and prayed silently for several minutes. Every move the mother made was prayerful.

Foreshadowings of her life's mission came to here even as a young girl in Yugoslavia. She was enthralled with stories of missionaries living in Bengal, India, the home state of Calcutta. By the time she was twelve she had become convinced that she should dedicate her life to God. She left home when she was eighteen, became a nun when she was twenty-one, and took her solemn vows when she was twenty-seven. When she was thirty-six she experienced the "call within the call" while traveling on a train to a convent in Darjeeling,

India. "I was to leave the convent and help the poor while living among them. It was an order. To fail would have been to break the faith," she recounted. She adopted Indian citizenship when she was thirty-eight years old, at the same time she began her missionary work in the slums of Calcutta.

Her work with the poorest of the poor did not come without challenges. In her diary she recounts that she had no income and had to beg for food and supplies. When she was first beginning her mission, she experienced doubt, loneliness, and the temptation to return to cloistered convent life.

The yoga group that had traveled to meet her moved closer. After a long period of time spent with each of the patients, the mother drifted into a much smaller room. Here, she gathered with all those who had come to see her. Softly she asked if we were pilgrims and which country we came from. Her talk with guests was much briefer. Her work was elsewhere. She talked about the spiritual rules of her order of nuns, and pointed to a sign on the wall behind her. I asked her what she would like to convey to us. She answered simply "Be good citizens of our country." Thirty years later I still ask myself, What did she mean by that statement? Did she perhaps know something we didn't, or see a future we couldn't see at the time?

Her talk ended with a reading on a little card she gave to each guest: "We think sometimes that poverty is only being hungry, naked, and homeless. The poverty of being unwanted, unloved, and uncared for is the greatest poverty. We must start in our own homes to remedy this kind of poverty."

Perseverance, courage, and will dominated Mother Teresa's efforts throughout her life. It wasn't until September 4, 2016 that the Catholic Church recognized her as a saint, nearly twenty years after her death in 1997. There is a saying that one moment in the presence of a saint can be your raft over the ocean of delusion. We are never too young or too old to visit saintly people. They remind us of our higher selves. Their stories give us the daring to live our own lives more heroically. And their very vibration can change us.

There is another way to help the world. We can send our healing prayers and thoughts to others. The fourth stage of yoga is the most powerful time of life. Everything we've learned, all our yoga meditation comes to fruition as each one of us, in a unique way, becomes like Mother Teresa, sharing our very vibration with those in need. The suffering, the refugees, and the homeless all need love. There is another group that rarely gets noticed that also needs our love and prayers. These are the prisoners who are incarcerated for life, unwanted, living their life behind bars. Many of us write to prisoners and pray for their well-being. It is a job that only the Divine will appreciate—our selfless prayers for those in deepest need throughout the planet.

There are numerous healing prayer networks throughout the world, organizations and churches that will pray for those in need. There can never be too many of us meditating together, praying together, sending out love.

"I see God in every human being. When I wash the leper's wounds, I feel I am nursing the Lord himself. Is it not a beautiful experience?"

—Mother Teresa of Calcutta, from a statement in 1977*

---

* As quoted in *Concise Oxford Dictionary of Quotations* (2011) by Susan Ratcliffe, p. 373.

CHAPTER 26

Yogis in Transition

Elders are healing and happy at a new home for yogis in transition.

As a friend of ours neared ninety, it became more difficult for her to get around, to drive and care for herself. As we age our world often becomes smaller; we may now do less than we did before. When she moved into Ananda House, located outside of Portland, Oregon, things were different. The personal attention, love, and healthy vegetarian meals she received at Ananda House gave her a dramatic boost of energy; her experience there was transformative in many ways.

At ninety she still sang in the choir in the Laurelwood yoga community and continued to engage in gardening activities there. On my last visit to see her, we sat in her room at Ananda House. She showed me watercolor paintings she had been working on—as lovely as ever, even in her very last years. I looked at her closely: "I love you, Gyandevi." Giving me a beautiful smile, she looked me in the eye: "I love you, too." She had the energy of a little girl, innocent and full of joy.

A similar transformation came to another elderly woman in Ananda House. She herself was not a yogi, but her daughter was. Her daughter told me that her mother had always been introverted and shy. After she'd been at Ananda House a few months she began to change. She began smiling more, talking with others and having fun. She was feeling much happier about life.

The leaders respond to difficulties the residents may have in their emotional lives—how to get along with others or how to battle depression. In a sharing circle everyone is invited to speak freely. Hanuman, Ananda House's co-director, used the forum of the sharing circle to speak openly of such challenges facing the residents, and would offer loving and creative solutions, ways to heal moods and bring more positivity.

Yoga provides a gentle way for older people to rise out of depression. As their world begins to shrink, older people may focus more and more on their own problems and worries. By giving them ways to refocus their energy into helping others or improving their own moods, yoga helps them forget their problems.

The positive effects of yoga can be enhanced by combining postures with positive affirmations. Also healing are simple ways to serve—reading to children, giving love to a dog or cat—anything that gives a feeling of making a contribution.

What is so striking about this house is the people who run it—a man trained as a hospice nurse and his wife, both of whom have lived the teachings of yoga for many years. It was Swami Kriyananda's sincere desire to see many little transition ashrams like Ananda House spring up in the future. He named these ashrams "Evening Hospice"—places where an elder's spiritual life is acknowledged and supported by loving caregivers.

In the evening, to keep the residents' spirits uplifted and focused on the Divine, beautiful chants and music are played at Ananda House.

Also refreshing at Ananda House is the quiet—no television sets blaring newscasts and sports. Instead, residents have daily schedules of yoga, meditation, music, chanting, as well as a variety of healthy, uplifting, and sattwic activities.

Residents are encouraged to work in the onsite organic vegetable gardens or to care for the botanical gardens that surround the house. Those who are able take walks around the neighborhood, take trips to the library, or to concerts with elevating music. For those who are housebound, friends and volunteers come over and read to them. Children from the Portland Living Wisdom School often visit, as do young people in the nearby Karma Yoga program. These visits bring an intergenerational community feel to the house.

The house for yogis in transition also has a training course for those wanting to create their own Evening Hospice. Guests can visit and learn; they can also attend one of the Seva workdays when elders and others work together to beautify the grounds and gardens that surround the house.

Yoga philosophy and support for elders are offered at Ananda House following Swami Kriyananda's core principles for Evening Hospice:

Twelve Precepts for Evening Hospice

1. To face the past.

2. To relinquish attachments.

3. To accept past errors without regret as simple facts, trying to see that it was God, through their imperfect understanding, Who did it all.

4. To release the grip of ego-consciousness.

5. To release, one by one, every desire and attachment into the supreme Bliss.

6. To offer every regret into God's love and Infinite Consciousness.

7. To forgive past hurts and betrayals.

8 To give out universal love to everyone, even to so-called enemies.

9. o help them see that everyone is motivated, however misguidedly by the same soul-craving for Satchitdananda (ever-existing, ever-conscious, ever-new bliss).

10. To concentrate on Infinity.

11. To practice devotion.

12. To learn to overcome fear by realizing that we are not this body.

CHAPTER 27

Con Te Partirò

For in and out, above, about, below,

'Tis nothing but a Magic Shadow-show,

Play'd in a Box whose Candle is the Sun,

Round which we Phantom Figures come and go.

— *The Rubaiyat of Omar Khyyam*
(translated by Edward FitzGerald), quatrain 46

ONE MORNING I STEPPED out of our cottage, closed the door, and moved down the trail to the Meditation Retreat office.

Something stirring in the pines, what was it?

Looking up, I saw that the wind was ruffling branches more vigorously than usual. A few steps more, I stopped and spun around, the pine needles beneath me crackling like the snapping of a thousand fingers.

What was that sound and where was it coming from? Was it a bird screeching, a couple talking? Was it a wildcat pursuing its prey?

I froze and listened. The Meditation Retreat was remote, isolated from normal human activity. It was too late in the morning for wildcats. I turned my head to the east.

Floating to my ears on the tip of a zephyr was a melody straight from the Teatro dell'Opera di Roma.

I looked down the hill, my eyes and ears focusing on the little *kutir*, a yurt two hundred feet below me. Music was coming through the trees, and though the words I heard were Italian, my heart tried to understand them. I couldn't stop listening. It was Andrea Bocelli, chanting the soulful "Con Te Partirò" ("Time to Say Goodbye"), with his irrepressible tenor.

My mind looked inside the *kutir* where the elderly retreat master was stepping about gracefully, his arms embracing the formless air in what felt like a Viennese wedding waltz. He was dressed in white tails made of graceful silk, a cheerful bowtie fastened at his neck. His snowy hair flowed behind him in a gentle wave that turned up before it reached his shoulders.

High in the pines, a trio of violins swooped down to play in the orchestra. Two cellos answered, and, levitating above his roof, astral fingers played the French horn. The entire Yuba River Gorge was filled up with the voice and the orchestra.

My own thoughts danced with him, the gentle mentor who used no words. His eyes were gazing through me with deep compassion, as if I didn't exist. I had learned more from living in close proximity to him than from a lifetime of lectures.

His instruction was always brief, coming mainly through his look, his energy, and his consciousness. His home was a red yurt hanging precariously over the steep river canyon. A small sign hung from the roof of his porch: *Satya Mandala.*

The universe started and stopped within his one-room geometric dome. A large painting of Yogananda drank up half the space and captured all who entered, the great yogi in orange robes, sitting in meditation posture, staring lovingly at his chela as he danced through morning chores.

His furniture was clean but worn, simple, straightforward. A small futon bed was folded up as a couch, pushed consciously to the side for his morning yoga and meditation.

This was the home of Satya, the eldest member of our Meditation Retreat community. I smiled inwardly, relaxed, drinking in the morning serenade.

Though Nakula and I were the official retreat leaders and also ran the college, Satya was very much a leader in his own right: an honored energy infusing and blessing the retreat as a whole. Now in his eighties, he could no longer attend to the worldly details that younger members of the community were good at. His wealth was his spiritual wisdom, and the deep knowledge of humankind that lives in a soul who is truly humble and of service to all.

Those who lived here, and the guests who came for seclusion and renewal, received the fruits of his many years of dedication to yoga meditation. His energy was in the ether, intangible, silent yet ever present.

His clothing was simple. He seemed to have only one sweater, brahmachari gold and with a rather large hole. On one level I wanted to darn the hole; to swipe it from him. On a deeper level I held back: there was something spiritually beautiful about his nonattachment to outward garb.

This morning, I knew he was dancing.

I surveyed the landscape on the cliff below me. Sitting on the broad deck behind Satya's kutir was a sturdy chaise lounge he used for his morning sun bath. On most days he took his prescribed twenty minutes of sun as he would a fresh-squeezed vegetable juice, gratefully and with enjoyment.

Beyond the deck were layer upon layer of pine forests, spreading out to the horizon in multidimensional shades of green.

Above me, a grey squirrel, commander of its tree, ran fifty feet up and stopped, glaring at me, his tail rudder hanging straight down, his energy gathered in a coiled spring, his eyes watching my every move. He held something in his tiny paws.

I continued to watch the vision below. Satya had moved onto the deck, his white tails fluttering. Physically, he was the ideal yogi. His dancing ability lent him a natural agility that extended to the various pretzel poses. Though his later years were spent at this remote seclusion retreat, in his earlier years he had been a sailor in the merchant marine and a dance instructor—a colorful background to his life in the forest.

The Meditation Retreat is one of only a few places that remind me of India's Himalayas. Located about five miles from the main yoga community, the retreat was the original location of the community.

Here was the abode of Satya, the original yoga master at the retreat in the late nineteen-sixties. Though Satya rarely spoke, he always had a warm greeting for any visitor or resident. His life during the stage of Sannyas was extremely simple. He would come to the temple for morning meditations, take a daily walk for exercise (usually out to Bald Mountain), and every now and then he'd have a visitor. When, occasionally, we'd have tea together, Satya would share his insights into the deeper teachings of yoga.

Right before our family moved from Ananda Village up through the foothills to the Meditation Retreat, the property was undergoing extensive brush clearing. The land was covered in wild Manzanita bushes, gnarled and the size of small trees, and a serious fire hazard. A walker often couldn't see the path to the temple or to the common dome. Ram, in earlier life a college football player, was helping to clear it away. Others came to help remove branches from the trees. Soon the land was covered in enormous burn piles, each one the size of a Safeway truck.

The Vedic fire ceremonies I'd seen had been fairly small, a few sticks in a wok. The power of the fire ceremony comes through the chanting of mantras together with a visualization: the participants are burning up seeds of karma from previous incarnations that are lodged in the astral spine.

The burn piles became a source of entertainment and a greatly expanded ceremony. Satya loved taking care of burn piles. Armed with heavy-duty tools, retreat staff and volunteers, men and women alike, joined Satya in his revelry. All were dressed in their dirtiest clothing; after a day of the burn piles, we were covered with ashes—we looked like Shiva's lost monks.

For the yogi, Shiva represents the manifestation of all that we cannot see, the unseen consciousness, the universal breath of all that is. As such, Shiva is the guardian of the four stages of yoga, the hidden energy behind the manifest.

Legend says Shiva lives in the forest, far away from human turbulence. Nothing can disturb either his inner peace or his careful resolve. He is not bothered by social standing, power, or worldly influences.

During our burn pile gatherings, the retreat became a home for Shiva. In his own way, Satya was serving Shiva as he tended the great fires as they burned up the tangles of brush that had been home to rakshasas*—both in the forest and in our minds. By the power of his devotion, Satya helped us all transform the burning of great piles of brush into a Vedic ceremony to purify the land and drive away all darkness.

In his home in Crystal Hermitage, Swami Kriyananda has a large brass statue of Nataraj, the dancing Shiva.

When we started the college at the Meditation Retreat in 2002, Satya became our biggest supporter. Now, well into his eighties, he was still a master of ballroom dancing. I asked him if he would teach dance to our college students. He was completely silent and didn't answer me.

A few days later he came right up to me and said, "Nischala, can we borrow that Nataraj statue from Swami's apartment? I want to use it for our dance class."

Satya placed the Nataraj statue, which was about four feet tall, high up on a table, as if Shiva himself were watching the dance class.

Pointing to the Nataraj, Satya told the students, "This is your instructor: Shiva is always centered, his energy deep in the spine. This is how you must learn to dance, from that center of inner calmness."

We all loved to watch Satya dance. He was part hermit, part yogi, part elegant gentleman. Sometimes, for a dance performance, he would dress in a tuxedo, just to show us that he wasn't bothered by outward roles and appearances. Swami Kriyananda told several of us who worked with young people that he wanted boys to learn to dance, that it would help them become more balanced and move gracefully through life's trials.

On the dance floor Satya became the dancing Shiva. His spine was always straight, his gaze inward, detached as though floating in some other world.

The Nataraja is Shiva as Lord of the Dance, representing rhythm and harmony of life. Nataraja is Shiva in his expanded role as creator, preserver, and destroyer, maintaining the continuous cycle of time, the four stages of

---

* Rakshasas are legendary demons in Vedic lore.

yoga, the four cycles of the yugas, and the Days and Nights of Brahma (the existence and dissolution of the physical universe).

The energy released by Shiva's dance makes his long matted locks fly in all directions; representing the boundless energy of the cycles of life and death. Shiva is the patron god of yoga.

Satya passed six months before my teacher. I led an astral ascension ceremony for him; a ceremony that my teacher, Swami Kriyananda, had written for souls transitioning from earth to the astral realms.

We all loved to watch Satya dance.

The following poem is often read following the Astral Ascension Ceremony.

Thou and I Are One

Thy cosmic life and I are one.
Thou art the Ocean, I am the wave;
 We are one.
Thou art the Flame, I am the spark;
 We are one.
Thou art the Flower, I am the fragrance.
 We are one.
Thou art the Father, I am Thy child;
 We are one.

Thou art the Beloved, I am the lover;
 We are one.
Thou art the Lover, I am the beloved;
 We are one.
Thou art the Song, I am the music;
 We are one.
Thou are the Spirit, I am all nature;
 We are one.
Thou art my Friend, I am Thy friend;
 We are one.

Thou art the Master, I am Thy servant;
    We are one.
Thou art the Mother, I am Thy son;
    We are one.
Thou art the Master, I am Thy disciple;
    We are one.
Thou art the Ocean, I am the drop;
    We are one.

Thou art all Laughter, I am a smile;
    We are one.
Thou art the Light, I am the atom;
    We are one.
Thou art Consciousness, I am the thought;
    We are one.
Thou art Eternal Power, I am strength;
    We are one.

Thy peace and I are one.
Thy joy and I are one.
Thy wisdom and I are one.
Thy love and I are one.
That is why Thou and I are one.
Thou and I were one, and Thou and I will be one evermore.[*]

(The ceremony closes by all rising, raise hands, and sending blessings and love to the departed.)

---

[*] Paramhansa Yogananda, *Whispers from Eternity* (Nevada City, California: Crystal Clarity Publishers, 2008), 199–200.

CHAPTER 28

The Rishi

The single goal of the fourth stage of yoga is moksha, *liberation.*

IT WAS AFTERNOON WHEN we began preparations for a visit to Dehra Dun in the Himalayan foothills.

Nakula and I were leading a group of college students on pilgrimage to northern India. We would be meeting Swami Jnanananda Giri, now in his fourth stage of yoga, and with much to share with our college.

His experience with yoga began when he was twenty-three and living in Switzerland. The day he received a copy of *Autobiography of a Yogi* was on March 7, 1952—the very day on which Yogananda entered *mahasamadhi*, a great yogi's conscious death. On this day Jnanananda set off on foot for India—and was never again to leave that holy ground.

Jnanananda (pronounced "Gyan-ananda") followed the traditional guide-lines presented by his guru, Swami Atmananda, a disciple of Swami Kebalananda, Yogananda's saintly Sanskrit tutor whose story is told in *Autobiography of a Yogi*.

The swami had suggested we bathe in the Ganges to purify ourselves, in keeping with traditional Vedic guidance for those wishing to visit holy people.

In higher civilizations, bodies of water are considered living entities. Rivers are seen as goddesses, and even ponds have their own sacred energy.

Environmentally aware countries such as New Zealand now call their rivers sacred. America will in time move in the same direction as we become aware of how vitally important our waters are.

For someone raised in India, the custom of taking a dip in the holy waters of the Ganges is ingrained. As a Westerner, I felt squeamish before my first experience, in 1987. *Dunk my whole body into a freezing, fast moving river three times?*

My mind was wondering whether I would be able to tie my sari on correctly for the ceremonial dip. On one of my earliest trips to India, as I was walking the crowded streets, I suddenly felt the entire contraption begin to slowly disengage. Once so gracefully draped around my shoulder and arm, the sari had become twisted into a mass that had snagged itself on my backpack. With every step I took, it unraveled. By the time I made it back to our lodging I had acres of cloth stuffed in the front of my pants, loose ends hanging everywhere.

Indians of many faiths view the purifying Ganges River as holy. Spun from the heavenly realms of Brahmaloka, the mystical river is said to travel to earth from the abode of Lord Shiva, deep in the Himalayas. Lord Shiva is said to keep the Ganges safe in his hair, infusing the river with his blessings as he lets her gradually flow down through the Himalayas.

For our ceremonial dip in the river I had decided to wear a white Punjabi outfit with pants and tunic. My husband Nakula, who must surely have been Indian in a recent incarnation, was perfectly relaxed in his dhoti as he walked to the banks of the Ganges. Patiently he waited for the right moment to say a prayer, bowed his head, and submerged elegantly into the glacial water. I sank down next to him and felt the water cover my face and head. A tingling feeling overcame me. The water seemed to have become droplets of radiant light, penetrating my aura and sending silent blessings. While my husband continued to immerse himself, I finished my dip and carefully backed out of the river.

We began our convoy to Dehra Dun in several of the old Ambassador taxis prevalent throughout India. Roads in India are a mystery to the linear

Western mind. Traffic flows in no set pattern, and repeatedly has to dodge a variety of obstacles, including animals, rickshaws, and ancient vehicles. Our driver pressed down on the accelerator and piloted around several large white Brahma bulls, a motorized rickshaw and an oncoming bus we missed by inches, the roar of motors accompanied by blaring horns.

The adrenalin of driving this way, combined with the baptism by water, had a fascinating effect.

We stopped midway for lunch at a South Indian café. Joining us for the occasion was Swami Bodhichitananda, the "Surfer Swami" as he was affectionately known by our college students. All smiles, Swami insisted we wash our hands, then ushered us quickly into tables. He was American, seemed younger than most swamis, kept his head shaved and wore orange robes according to the custom of the Sivananda ashram, where he received his monastic vows from the late Swami Chidananda Saraswati. At one time he had been a sannyasi/monk with Self-Realization Fellowship in California, and now considered Swami Jnanananda his Kriya Yoga guru.

"Before we get to Dehra Dun, we need to stop and get some food and prasad for Swamiji," he said. He explained that Jnanananda was a traditional sannyasi who depended on others to care for him. I asked him what we should get. "Some good bread, jam, nuts, and fruits," he replied.

In India, sannyasis who renounce the world traditionally wandered as mendicants, relying on donations from others. In earlier time they traveled on foot; modern-day sannyasis travel by vehicle, even in airplanes. A traditional sannyasi has no fixed abode. They must not be bound by any one place, but must see the whole world as their home. Such a one gives up everything and lives by God's will and grace alone.

We all moved more slowly after lunch. Our taxi convoy outside also seemed half asleep. We boarded our ancient vehicle. Groping for seatbelts, I remembered these older models were unequipped. I had a flashback of the American movie I'd been shown as a fifteen-year-old on the virtues of seat belts. If I were to fly through the air like a plastic dummy, better it be while visiting a saint.

Our driver, seeming to catch my thought, smiled at us in the rear view mirror. A small statue of the Hindu goddess Durga sat on his dashboard, gracefully riding her tiger side-saddle, an array of weapons cascading from her eight arms, esoteric symbols of such virtues as courage, detachment, and righteousness. The driver swerved, barely missing a young man pedaling a bicycle. I closed my eyes, ducked, and grabbed Nakula's arm.

Approaching Dehra Dun, we saw above what appeared to be a storefront grocery hosting a simple sign with the word "sweet." The taxi turned into a dusty space next to a few old motorcycles, again narrowly missing someone, this time an elderly man sitting on his haunches tending a cup of tea. Our driver turned off the engine, the old metal shaking and wheezing. He tossed a few words of Hindi to the man taking tea; they smiled at each other like old friends.

Inside, we hunted for gifts for Swami Jnanananda. Sweets are offered as prasad, a symbol of the seeker's devotion and gratitude to the Divine. Once this offering has been blessed by a Divine channel, it is considered sacred and passed around to devotees.

"Oh, that looks good," a student was pointing to fried donut holes floating in syrup.

The grocery store clerk packed up a large box of the syrupy confection, wrapped it with paper, tied the box securely with colored string, and handed it to Nakula with a big smile. "*Very* good," the man said, "Very . . ." The clerk paused and smiled again, "*Sweet.*"

It was late afternoon by the time we reached Jnanananda's home, which was actually the home of one of his devotees, now turned into a small ashram. The swami greeted us with welcoming smiles and chatter. His energy appeared locked in his inner spine. There were no wasted words or movements. His white beard was untrimmed and abundant, his long hair pulled up into the tiny topknot of the rishi.

The topknot, worn during the day, is meant to stimulate the frontal lobes of the brain, the area engaged in meditation and other states of deeper spiritual awareness. The rishis let their hair down in the evening to allow it to spread out and capture the energy of the moon and the ether.

Many advanced yogis never cut their hair or beards; the fine hairs are said to be transmitters and receivers of subtle and psychic energy. It is further believed that if you refrain from cutting your hair for three years, it will grow to its natural length, giving the yogi increased subtle mental powers, patience, and energy.

The prana from the ether that sensitive rishis are able to capture nourishes and sustains the body without physical food. This is how yogis live hundreds of years. In *Autobiography of a Yogi,* Yogananda writes of Giri Bala, the non-eating saint. From the time she was twelve she never took food; she lived instead on the finer energies of the air and sunlight and from the cosmic power which recharged her body through the medulla oblongata, at the base of the brain.

To shave one's head also has a yogic rationale, one with parallels to gardening. Often yogis shave their heads on Shivaratri, one day before the new moon in February. A new moon is also considered an auspicious time to plant seeds in a garden. Just as pruning a tree concentrates energy in the pruned area, so does shaving the head allow energy to move towards the two highest chakras in the head—the sixth chakra, at the point between the eyebrows, and the seventh chakra, the lotus or crown chakra at the top of the head.

On later visits to Jnanananda, we often found his white hair worn pulled up Indian-style inside a turban—not the precisely wound and tightly tucked turban worn by Sikhs, but loose and casual, coming apart in a few areas.

The swami led us around the outside of his small ashram, beginning near the front and walking in a clockwise direction, circumambulating it three times, as Hindu devotees do at shrines of their faith. The building was round and two-storied, camouflaged behind the plant creepers that covered it—the ashram seemed to be hiding in a jungle. The courtyard garden was filled with trees and plants, interwoven with soft dirt paths. Some of the larger trees had sitting benches tucked next to them.

"You should have your college students learn to walk barefoot on the earth," Jnanananda urged. His accent was Swiss. "Doing so will allow them to connect to the earth's magnetic field in a more profound way. They will learn subtle truths through this experience."

He took us to a tree in his garden and sat lotus style on a bench, pulling his back right up next to the tree: "This tree has healed me of sickness many times." He demonstrated how to draw energy from the tree by placing one's left hand behind the body and against the tree, and how then to channel healing energy from the tree into your body by placing the right hand across the heart chakra.

"You should try this. Trees can be powerful healing instruments with much more knowledge of our needs than we are aware of." He suggested that we use only the healthiest of trees. "A healthy tree lovingly cared for can become our ally."

Jnanananda had spent his entire adult life close to nature.

Rishis of Vedic India lived in remote forests and in harmony with wild animals. In no other part of the ancient world are nonviolence and compassion for animals so pervasive. Even the Buddha's compassion stemmed from the spiritual ethos of India.

"In higher ages the rishis use trees to communicate across long distances. Trees are noble beings, especially those that have been on earth for hundreds or thousands of years," he said.

Vanamali Devi once told us that the rishis considered the peepul tree holy because it's the only tree that emits oxygen throughout the night and day. Devotees who circumambulated this tree received the benefit of its steady output of oxygen. The rishis also revered the peepul tree, Vanamali explained, as one of the expressions of the divine energy infusing all trees and plants, as a focus to awaken understanding that every aspect of nature is worthy of worship.

Once inside his ashram we met Swami Jnanananda's disciple, host, and caretaker, a congenial Indian woman named Maitreya—she told us how the swami had come to inherit the small dog he was holding:

"One day a taxi showed up at our door with a small dog in the backseat. The taxi had been driven from Delhi with no instructions other than to bring the dog here. Though he had no interest in pets, Swamiji decided there must be some reason for this odd occurrence and decided to keep the dog."

The dog that had mysteriously arrived in the taxi was a small Lhasa Apso, a breed that originated near the sacred city of Lhasa, in Tibet, where they were kept as temple or monastery dogs. There are legends that when a monk, priest or lama dies, if one has not reached nirvana, they will be reincarnated as one of these sacred temple dogs.

If someone in our group moved, "Dharma" would bark and growl, not so much viciously, as to make a statement: the kind of warning bark commonly issued by small dogs with bangs in their eyes and property to defend.

Our hosts invited us into the front room, which served as a small temple, with room for about twenty-five people tightly packed. We sat on the floor, on stools, and on the elaborate staircase.

With Dharma watching our every move, we knew now to hold very still. If one of us moved or became restless in thought, he would bark loudly.

Jnanananda spoke of the yoga principle, "What comes of itself, let it come"—we must embrace everything that comes to us and look inside to understand why. The swami said he felt intuitively that the dog was a disciple who had died and reincarnated as this dog, specifically to be close to him and protect him. The dog disciple, we can assume, was blessed by his service to his guru/master.

While traveling in India many years ago, I found a book with a strange paragraph explaining that both Lahiri Mahayasa and Swami Sri Yukteswar were working on ways to help animals reincarnate from the animal to the human stage: It was to the dog's or the cat's benefit to become domesticated. By "domesticated," I'm assuming the animal would live mainly indoors, not roaming free, chasing and killing other animals. Living closely with humans, especially with spiritually minded humans, would help these animals to evolve.

As I listened to the swami's gentle discourse, I reflected on our own pet. Many of us living as householders in our community keep cats. The community does not allow dogs to roam free because of the likelihood of their forming packs to chase deer. When our son, Rama, was about seven he began asking me for a baby brother or sister to play with. Not wishing to have more than one child, I prayed to Divine Mother for a solution to my son's loneliness. Several months later a young kitten came darting across our small deck; the kitten seemed to have simply manifested from the nearby forest. I watched it, commenting on its beauty, but quickly lost sight of it as the little creature disappeared.

A few weeks later, Rama and I saw a group of cats congregating near Hansa Temple. One young cat left the group and ran right towards us. When Rama opened our car door, it jumped into the back seat. It was the same kitten we'd seen earlier running across our deck. Rama had a new friend. I began searching for notices of a lost kitten. I called around, put up a notice with a photo, but no one responded. The cat appeared to had been well taken care of, was already neutered and quite affectionate. We waited and watched, and after a few weeks, decided to keep it.

Several times during the night the cat would steeplechase onto beds, furniture, and foreheads as if being pursued by wild animals. Once I saw it run straight towards a mirror, look at its own reflection, then dance sideways like a crab, fur puffed up as though it had been electrocuted. They have their own methods of entertainment.

In the presence of this saintly swami, we all became quiet and reflective. I could feel his highly sensitive nature. Neither the swami—nor his dog—missed a movement or a thought.

Jnanananda was silent during much of our time with him. When he did speak, the words came out in a measured way, his Swiss accent adding to the preciseness of his speech: "Here is an important quote, remember it. 'If in wisdom's way you want to walk, five things observe with care, to whom you talk, of whom you talk, how, when, and where.'"

The room was silent. After a few minutes he continued, "This is a quote from Saint Mirdad,* said to be the guru of Noah." Silence reigned for several minutes until he spoke again: "So speak as if the world entire were but a single ear intent on hearing what you say."

---

* *The Book of Mirdad: The Strange Story of a Monastery Which Was Once Called the Ark* by Mikhail Naimy (First South Asian Edition 2006, Watkins Publishing, London, www.watkinspublishing.com).

On his altar was a large Shiva linga sitting inside a bowl, presumably to catch water or milk used to bathe it in ceremonies. A stick of incense burned, its gentle smoke rising. Red flowers were spread over the altar.

More silence. Then he said, "Yoga means to watch your breath." He paused. "To know your relationship to the breath and to give thanks to the breath, which many people don't ever do. I have met yogi practitioners who have been practicing over thirty years, but they forget to give thanks to the breath."

He waited a few moments. "And yet we all know that according to the Bible, when God created man, He was breathing His own breath into man." Again he paused. "It means the debt belongs to God."

At his side was an old harmonium.

Having lived most of my life in a yoga ashram in the West, I was well acquainted with the Indian harmonium used for chanting *bhajans* (devotional songs to God).

We listened to the swami as he played bhajans and sang.

It is said that sound is the sensory experience most influential on our consciousness. The experience of listening to the swami's chanting is difficult to describe. I've never seen anyone play the harmonium as he did. He was one with his instrument, the harmonium an extension of his being. His music brought us into his inner world—decades of solitude, meditation, and inner realization. When he was twenty-three he left behind a promising career as a musician. His life devoted to God was now blessing our group.

One of our students wanted to film him with a movie camera. Gently he raised his hand, demurring: "Take a photograph with your heart."

The swami explained further, "It was only when I met my guru that I understood—he told me: 'First look for God, then everything else will be given to you.'"

He asked us to play the harmonium. After hearing his exquisite playing, we sounded like school children learning to play the musical scale.

He asked us about our college, and looked at a photo of Machu Picchu in our brochure. After gazing at the photo for some time, he said he'd been there in a past life: then, looking directly at Nakula, he added, "And you were there too!" Nakula didn't know what to say. Looking closely into Nakula's eyes, the rishi softly spoke: "You think I'm joking. I'm not."

As our receptivity deepened, the rishi began to play with our hearts and minds.

Jnanananda was a man of slight build, not at all large or robust. In ordinary conversation, or when he played the harmonium, we reeled in the presence of such power. He put everything he had into the music, his body swaying, his chants suggesting fathomless states of wisdom.

To be a sannyasi means ultimately to end all worldly ties. The sannyasi abandons not society itself, but the entangling rituals of the social world. Many live in silence and seclusion, without fixed abode. Family, friends, material possessions—all these must eventually go, to allow the sannyasi the freedom to go deep in the Divine.

The single goal of the fourth stage of yoga is *moksha*, liberation. Liberation, for some sannyasis, means achieving union with the Divine, ideally without rebirth in a future life. For others, liberation means the experience of the highest samadhi. For still others, liberation means jivanmukta—Self-realization while they are still living.

In March 2015, as I was working on this chapter, I began to feel the desire to return to India. "We need to go back to see Swami Jnanananda," I made this plea to Nakula several times. A few months later we found through Swami Bodhichitananda that Swami Jnanananda had left his body, during the very time I had been writing his chapter.

Wishing to know more about Jnanananda's passing, I contacted Swami Bodhichitananda, as well as Ram Alexander and his wife Parvati, two disciples of Anandamoyi Ma we had met in India when traveling with the college. They told me his body had been laid to rest in a small temple near Simla.

During visits with our college Jnanananda sometimes gave me copies of his poetry or chapters from his autobiography. At one time the rishi had lived in caves in the foothills of the Himalayas above and around Rishikesh. In his autobiography, *Transcendent Journey*, he talks about his close friendship with two other swamis; the three would meet and occasionally roam together through the dense forests near Rishikesh and Hardwar:

"In their company I relished an inner attunement and a definite state of realization. Both these swamis were of the most joyous disposition because of their closeness to God. Discussions often brought about outbursts of merriment with peals of laughter. I was indeed privileged to sport in the presence of Nirvendananda and Bhumananda. To me, it was as if these two were the very manifestation of my own soul. Such friendship endures. But with the passage of time, the outer picture in this world changes constantly."*

This excerpt is taken from "Call of the Heart," a poem written by Jnanananda Giri:

"Snow is slowly falling over the forest-clad slopes of the great Himalaya. Like a shower of heavenly nectar, these white flakes, soft as cotton, float down from the Eternal Above to touch the earth where they dissolve. God-experience in the sublime spiritual atmosphere of the dreamy snow-covered Himalaya is the fulfilment of my inmost longing. How could I resist contemplating on that Supreme Being that created all this beauty!

"Diving deep within into my heart, day after day, I approached an ever-present silence that reveals the true glory of the soul. Such must be the blessed moments when yogis enter the transcendental meditation on the Absolute. One's whole being melts in bliss and love. Oh Lord, how wonderful!

"The realm of God is in the depth and vastness of the soul! The soul, spread out as it were, appears as divine nature to the all-penetrating vision of the seer whose individuality merges with the One Existence. Frozen by the frost of inscrutable powers of faith, the Eternal Absolute vibrates with creative energy and ideation, therewith fully covering the imagination of the Cosmic Dreamer.

"Deep within the infinite heart of man lies the divine desire that projects phenomenal creations as willed by Him in unceasing rhythm, the transcendental sport of the Divine—a mere play evolving from the intelligent, harmonious source of primal ideation in the causal body of man, *the heart!*"

---

* Swami Jnanananda, *Transcendent Journey.* Jnanananda gave a digital copy of his autobiography to Nakula and me years ago. We visited him many times with the college and he would sometimes give me poetry he had written or pages from his manuscript. I believe he knew I would someday write this book and include his story and writings. Om Tat Sat.

HEAVENLY ABODES & ASTRAL PLANES

HIGHER ASTRAL PLANES	Satyaloka (Sphere of God)	
	Tapoloka (Universal Spirit)	**Hiranyaloka
*Premabhava	Janaloka (Spiritual Reflection)	
	Maharloka (Sphere of Atoms)	
	Bhuvarloka (Sphere of Fine Matter)	
EARTH PLANE	Bhuloka (Sphere of Gross Matter)	

* Premabhava residing on the abode of spiritual reflection

LOWER ASTRAL PLANES

** In *Autobiography of a Yogi,* Sri Yukteswar said he was living on Hriyanaloka, an illumined astral planet that no one can enter unless they have advanced to the highest state of nirbikalpa samadhi. Its location is unknown; perception requires the highest state of samadhi. The faculty of Ananda University, while exploring Sri Yukteswar's writings, have created this simple one-dimensional chart to explain an astral world that is unfathomable. We do know that the rishis describe seven "lokas," or stages of creation. These are described in sutra 27 of Sri Yukteswar's book, *The Holy Science.*

CHAPTER 29

Death and the Astral Planes

"As certain redwood trees outlive most trees by millenniums, or as some yogis live several hundred years . . . , so some astral beings live much longer than the usual span of astral existence. Visitors to the astral world dwell there for a longer or shorter period in accordance with the weight of their physical karma, which draws them back to earth within a specified time."

—Sri Yukteswar explaining the astral planes in the
chapter titled "The Resurrection of Sri Yukteswar" in
Autobiography of a Yogi

THE AFTERLIFE IS A haven, and at the same time simply another journey within the great cycles of birth and rebirth. In whatever stage of life we find ourselves, we have work to do to prepare for the final exam of death.

During the final stage of yoga we are confronted with any accumulated attachments that we have not yet released. Attachments come in many forms—relationships we still cling to (even those with our pets), our cars, our possessions, our fleeting status, our earthly passions. Our spiritual duty is not so much to get rid of things and feelings as to learn not to be attached to them.

213

The goal of life is to merge back into God. As Swami Jnanananda said, "Diving deep within into my heart, day after day, I approached an ever-present silence that reveals the true glory of the soul. Such must be the blessed moments when yogis enter the transcendental meditation on the Absolute. One's whole being melts in bliss and love. Oh Lord, how wonderful!"

My teacher, Swami Kriyananda often reminded us, "We must learn to live each day as if it is our last, because we never know when we will go."

When a close friend was nearing her final transition, she made a specific request: her breathing prevented her practicing Kriya Yoga meditation herself, she asked me to do Kriya for her as I sat by her bedside, so that she could bask in the holy Kriya vibration.

Other souls in transition have found comfort, courage, and inspiration in listening to recordings of sacred music—*Life Mantra* (formerly titled *Chant of the Angels*), the AUM chant, the Maha Mantra, or the auspicious Gayatri or Mahamritunjaya Mantras.*

On the *Life Mantra* album, a heavenly choir sings two simple phrases—"God is Love, God is Joy"—the essence of the yogi's quest. The singers are all yogis. While recording the album, some choir members had experiences of angels appearing to them.

Yogananda describes the death process in detail. "When the ordinary person approaches death, usually his whole body becomes paralyzed, just as part of your body sometimes 'goes to sleep.' When your foot goes to sleep, you see it, and you know that it is yours, but you cannot move or use it. So, at the approach of death, most people feel an entire paralysis, or a going-to-sleep state of the entire body—limbs, muscles, and even internal organs, including heart, lungs, and diaphragm.

"In the beginning, the dying person is conscious of the slow falling asleep of the muscles and limbs. When the heart begins to grow numb, there is a sense of suffocation, because without heart action the lungs cannot operate. This sense of suffocation is a little painful for about one to three seconds, and causes a great fear of death. Because souls reincarnate many times, and

---

* CDs of this music, composed and/or performed by Swami Kriyananda, are available through Crystal Clarity Publishers.

necessarily have to experience death in passing from an old body into the body of a little child, they retain the memory of this feeling of suffocation and pain at death. This memory of pain causes fear of death."*

Saints of many traditions have spoken about the afterlife review—a time when a condensed evaluation of all the good and bad actions of one's lifetime comes up in the mind of the dying person. This mental introspection is presented in a way that graphically helps the soul determine the kind of rebirth required in the next life.

Because hearing is the last physical sense to leave the body, the dying person can be helped by loving, uplifting words whispered, and OM (AUM) chanted softly in the right ear. Negative, hopeless comments such as "All is lost" or "She's going now" can damage the peace of the soul's transition. We don't know exactly when a soul will pass to the other side. Until the transition is complete, the soul retains a level of awareness of the earth plane. Many published accounts describe people coming back from "death" and remembering the exact words that were spoken after they had left their body.

The time of transition and soon afterwards is the time to offer prayers for the soul's quick ascension to the heavenly abodes. My teacher, Swami Kriyananda, wrote a lovely "astral ascension" ceremony, a ceremony we come together for within a few days of a friend's passing. It is an opportunity for families, friends, and loved ones to offer prayers and final goodbyes. In the Hindu tradition, the body is cremated as soon as possible after physical death so that the ascended soul sees the body burning, and knows not to try to "re-enter," but to pass on to the higher planes.

When a family member or a close friend has died suddenly, when an astral ascension ceremony is not immediately possible, our best service is to meditate and send light to the transitioning soul. The astral body may still be on a plane near the earth and so may need help moving up into the light of the higher planes. The departed being may be in confusion—trying to return to the physical body, trying be near loved ones. We can help the soul's journey into the light by visualizing that soul ascending towards the heavenly abodes.

---

* Paramhansa Yogananda, *Karma and Reincarnation* (Nevada City, California: Crystal Clarity Publishers, 2007), 57.

Yogis with a strong spiritual practice can be called on to send light to the soul struggling to reach the higher realms. It is best to continue praying and sending light to the departed soul for at least two weeks—even longer if intuition so guides those praying.

For my brother, who had a lonely life and not many friends, I prayed for his departed soul for an entire year, asking Yogananda and other great masters to see the inherent goodness of his soul and to help him ascend. I prayed for my mother for six months after her death. Tuning in to other transitions I have often intuited that the departed soul was in the right place, or even thriving in the heavenly realms.

We can also send prayers to friends and loved ones in the heavenly realms—to ask those ascended souls to help another departed soul or even ourselves. Highly evolved souls, especially who care deeply about us, may speak to us in secret ways. Angels do exist. We may speak lightly of them, but our souls remember these beings; we ourselves may have helped others in their transitions between lives. The greatest help for souls in transition comes from such great masters as Yogananda, Christ, Buddha, and Krishna.

The Vedas describe five to eight million lives in lower forms before a soul reaches human incarnation. Yogananda remembered his own lifetimes as far back as his life as a diamond. To live now as a human being means the soul has traveled a very long road to its return journey to freedom in God. The gift of human life is too precious to be cast aside in suicide, no matter how difficult the journey.

The life review that occurs after a person has died is a staging point, an opportunity to choose lessons to learn in the next life. Our final thoughts are enormously important to determining our next life's journey. It is for this same reason that the evolving soul should struggle against addiction and all worldly attachments, free itself of entanglements, forgive every past hurt with a forgiveness that goes even to ourselves, and go into the light with positive, blissful thoughts and love for God.

When Yogananda entered mahasamadhi on March 7, 1952, he consciously left his body by stopping his heart. He had said before that a heart attack was the easiest way to go, and the way he chose for his own exit. The great yogis may leave their bodies in widely varied ways. Lahiri Mahasaya announced his death beforehand. Yukteswar went while Yogananda was on holiday, then later appeared miraculously in the flesh to his disciple, at that time further schooling him in the nature of life on other planes. Yogananda exited the body while reading his poem "My India," a tribute in part to his life-long mission from Mahavatar Babaji to bring yoga to the West, and fulfillment of his own prophecy that he would leave his body speaking of "my America and my India."

When Gandhi died by assassination, his soul had long been fully prepared: In perfect accord with the simple lifestyle of this great leader, Gandhi left behind only his glasses, a copy of the Bhagavad Gita, a pair of wooden sandals, a cup, and the three "see-no-evil, hear-no-evil, speak-no-evil" monkeys. We each experience death according to our own karma.

Swami Kriyananda explained that some souls leave the body through the lower chakras, and some through the higher chakras, or through the third eye in the forehead. When a soul exits through the seventh, or "crown" chakra, that soul has achieved final liberation. Towards the end of his life, Kriyananda spoke often of what he called the "final exam" of death:

"What we want to do is finish this life on a high note. Keep your accounts clear. If you hurt someone, pray for that person, if you can't apologize directly. Cancel out your debts when you've been dishonest. If you cheated someone, give something away. We must realize that our home is in God, and that the goal of life is to merge back into God. This physical plane is the lowest of the planes of existence. We want to get out of this physical plane. So don't build attachments. When you go to bed at night, create a mental fire and cast into that fire all your longings and attachments, all your desires. Go through your heart daily . . . .like walking through the fields picking out burrs, try to feel that you're picking out the burrs in your heart—pick them out and throw them into the fire. You will find that you will feel very free.

"People can go suddenly. You don't know when you go to bed at night if you'll be gone in the morning. It's a wonderful practice to offer everything up; say 'God, it's not my world, it's Your world; I am not attached.' That is why the Bhagavad Gita stresses *nishkam karma*, action without desire for the fruits of action. We have to act in this world to be a success. We must do our best. We've come to the human level and we have the capacity to make a better world; we should do what we can to help other people and to make things beautiful.

"Some people have a negative attitude, thinking 'It's all a dream, so it won't matter, so why bother?' God put us here to be good stewards. There's a story about an Irish priest visiting a farmer. The priest said, 'Oh, what a beautiful family God has given you.' 'Oh what a beautiful home God has given you.' 'Oh, what a beautiful farm God has given you.' By this time, the farmer had had enough: 'Well, Father, you may be right, but you should have seen this farm when God had it all to Himself!' And so it is that we must do our best to work with God. He has given us the free will to be co-creators with Him. Although the end of life is death, nonetheless we should do our best; it's His world, not ours."

"What happens at death is that we leave our physical bodies behind but don't leave our consciousness behind; we take that with us. In that consciousness are lots of desires that may bring us back to this earth plane. For instance, if your desire is for a car, there are no cars in heaven, so you'll have to come back here. If your desire is to smoke, there are no cigarettes in heaven, so you'll have to come back here. If your desire is for money, fame, power, or sex, those desires will direct us back to this world.

"When the soul is ready to leave the body, the energy begins to withdraw from the senses, just as in sleep. Sleep, you might say is 'the little death.' In death, that energy withdraws more completely.

"When you leave your body all the intense pain you may have experienced during this life is gone. If you're burned at the stake, if people murder you, once you're out of your body there's no pain at all. There's a sense of great relief, great freedom; and in near-death experiences, people have found themselves looking down at their bodies. In that state when you are leaving, you can often still hear people talking . . . so what is said and communicated to one another, especially through doctors and nurses, caregivers, etc., is very important. As long as you are still near the world your senses are still perfectly clear. There is still the power of seeing, the power of hearing, the power of feeling.

"All of the senses are in the energy body and not just in the physical body. Deaf people, in their astral bodies, can hear perfectly. People who have been born blind, at death see perfectly. When you go into the other world, you're a free person. You'd like to stay there, but you have to come back if there are desires. Freedom is the goal."

In the realm of yoga there are few books that directly explain what happens in the astral planes or the afterlife. *Autobiography of a Yogi* offers the clearest, most thorough reference anywhere. In the chapter titled "The Resurrection of Sri Yukteswar," Yogananda listens as his guru schools him in the intricate and subtle states of awareness after death. Yogananda once told my teacher that Yukteswar wrote his book, *The Holy Science,* while in *nirbikalpa samadhi,* a state of true illumination in which a liberated yogi can see all of creation, as well as all people's thoughts from past, present, and future.

Visions are not necessarily a sign of spiritual advancement. Visions can come simply for the benefit of a spiritual aspirant who is in need of a sign, perhaps to encourage that person to develop spiritually.

Several builders creating a small temple dedicated to Lahiri Mahasaya at Ananda Village had spiritual experiences of the yoga masters blessing the temple during construction. One older gentleman saw a great beam of light, and with the beam of light an image of the great Kriya Yogi Lahiri Mahasaya, come down from above to illuminate the entire shrine.

Here at the Meditation Retreat a small group of people had just finished a sacred Kriya Yoga initiation. When they walked out of the Temple of Silence they saw Mahavatar Babaji meditating on a small hill above an underground room we now call the Babaji Cave. He was overlooking a spot where we were planning to develop a garden pool. This pool we have named Babaji Pool, dedicated to the deathless yogi.

The miraculous experiences that came to Yogananda, especially the resurrection of Sri Yukteswar and his detailed description of the astral planes—all these Yogananda has transmitted through *Autobiography of Yogi* in order to give aspiring yogis a glimpse into the vast realms beyond the limited earth plane. After his mahasamadhi, Yukteswar appeared to his disciple Yogananda in the flesh; Yukteswar described the nature of the astral and causal planes, and explained how and why souls reincarnate.

Yukteswar explains to Yogananda that though he has created a new body identical to his old one out of cosmic atoms, he is now living on an astral planet whose inhabitants are better able to meet his lofty standards than the inhabitants of the earth plane. On *Hiryanaloka*, Yukteswar is "aiding advanced beings to rid themselves of astral karma and thus attain liberation from astral rebirths."

"Unlike the spacial, three-dimensional physical world cognized only by the five senses, the astral spheres are visible by the all-inclusive sixth sense—intuition," Sri Yukteswar explains. "By sheer intuitional feeling, all astral beings see, hear, smell, taste and touch. They possess three eyes, two of which are partly closed. The third and chief astral eye, vertically placed on the forehead, is open."

Yogananda explained that, through his own perfect attunement to his guru, he received Yukteswar's communication in the forms of word-pictures and thought-transference. The following are a few more excerpts from "The Resurrection of Sri Yukteswar":

"Offspring are materialized by astral beings through the help of their cosmic will into specially patterned, astrally condensed forms. The recently physically disembodied being arrives in an astral family through invitation, drawn by similar mental and spiritual tendencies. . . .

"Joyous astral festivities on the higher astral planets like Hiranyaloka take place when a being is liberated from the astral world through spiritual advancement, and is therefore ready to enter the heaven of the causal world. On such occasions the Invisible Heavenly Father, and the saints who are merged in Him, materialize Themselves into bodies of Their own choice and join the astral celebration. In order to please His beloved devotee, the Lord takes any desired form. If the devotee worshiped through devotion, he sees God as the Divine Mother. To Jesus, the Father-aspect of the Infinite One was appealing beyond other conceptions. The individuality with which the Creator has endowed each of His creatures makes every conceivable and inconceivable demand on the Lord's versatility!

"Friends of other lives easily recognize one another in the astral world," Sri Yukteswar went on in his beautiful, flutelike voice. "Rejoicing at the immortality of friendship, they realize the indestructibility of love, often doubted at the time of the sad, delusive partings of earthly life.

"The intuition of astral beings pierces through the veil and observes human activities on earth, but man cannot view the astral world unless his sixth sense is somewhat developed. Thousands of earth-dwellers have momentarily glimpsed an astral being or an astral world."

Here is Sri Yukteswar's description of the high astral planet, Hiranyaloka: "The advanced beings on Hiranyaloka remain mostly awake in ecstasy during the long astral day and night, helping to work out intricate problems of cosmic government and the redemption of prodigal sons, earthbound souls. When the Hiranyaloka beings sleep, they have occasional dreamlike astral visions. Their minds are usually engrossed in the conscious state of highest nirbikalpa bliss. . . . Communication among the astral inhabitants is held entirely by astral telepathy and television."

Sri Yukteswar explains that astral beings intuitively recognize loved ones on other planes of existence: "Because every atom in creation is inextinguishably dowered with individuality, an astral friend will be recognized no matter what costume he may don."

Beyond the astral worlds lies the causal, here elucidated by Sri Yukteswar: "The span of life in the astral world is much longer than on earth. A normal advanced astral being's average life period is from five hundred to one thousand years, measured in accordance with earthly standards of time. . . .

"Causal desires are fulfilled by perception only. The nearly-free beings who are encased only in the causal body see the whole universe as realizations of the dreams-ideas of God; they can materialize anything and everything in sheer thought. Causal beings therefore consider the enjoyment of physical sensations or astral delights as gross and suffocating to the soul's fine sensibilities. Causal beings work out their desires by materializing them instantly. Those who find themselves covered only by the delicate veil of the causal body can bring universes into manifestation even as the Creator. Because all creation is made of the cosmic dream-texture, the soul thinly clothed in the causal has vast realizations of power,"* the great master concluded.

---

* Sri Yukteswar quoted on these pages: Paramhansa Yogananda, *Autobiography of a Yogi* (Nevada City, California: Crystal Clarity Publishers, 2005), 400, 403, 404–5, 407, 409.

Yogananda described the astral world as a realm in which whatever we can imagine can happen and is true. It is difficult to conceive with our limited human understanding the vast expanse of the universes that exist beyond our tiny speck of earth. The spiritual state of great masters is beyond human comprehension, just as the knowledge and abilities normal in the higher yugas are unfathomable to the earthbound mind. Our contemporary understanding of the universe from a physical and scientific perspective has long ages ago been surpassed by the profound wisdom of the Vedic masters.

"In order to please His beloved devotee, the Lord takes any desired form. If the devotee worshiped through devotion, he sees God as the Divine Mother. To Jesus, the Father-aspect of the Infinite One was appealing beyond other conceptions. The individuality with which the Creator has endowed each of His creatures makes every conceivable and inconceivable demand on the Lord's versatility!"

—Swami Sri Yukteswar, *Autobiography of a Yogi*

CHAPTER 30

Paramhansa Yogananda wrote this poem about the highest state of meditation—union with God—while riding the subway in New York City. He advised people to memorize the poem as a reminder of the goal of all spiritual striving.

Samadhi

Vanished the veils of light and shade,

Lifted every vapor of sorrow,

Sailed away all dawns of fleeting joy,

Gone the dim sensory mirage.

Love, hate, health, disease, life, death,

Perished these false shadows on the screen of duality.

Waves of laughter, scyllas of sarcasm, melancholic whirlpools,

Melting in the vast sea of bliss.

The storm of *maya* stilled

By magic wand of intuition deep.

The universe, forgotten dream, subconsciously lurks,

Ready to invade my newly-wakened memory divine.

I live without the cosmic shadow,

But it is not, bereft of me;
As the sea exists without the waves,
But they breathe not without the sea.
Dreams, wakings, states of deep *turia* sleep,
Present, past, future, no more for me,
But ever-present, all-flowing I, I, everywhere.
Planets, stars, stardust, earth,
Volcanic bursts of doomsday cataclysms,
Creation's molding furnace,
Glaciers of silent x-rays, burning electron floods,
Thoughts of all men, past, present, to come,
Every blade of grass, myself, mankind,
Each particle of universal dust,
Anger, greed, good, bad, salvation, lust,
I swallowed, transmuted all
Into a vast ocean of blood of my own one Being!
Smoldering joy, oft-puffed by meditation
Blinding my tearful eyes,
Burst into immortal flames of bliss,
Consumed my tears, my frame, my all.
Thou art I, I am Thou,
Knowing, Knower, Known, as One!
Tranquilled, unbroken thrill, eternally living, ever-new peace!
Enjoyable beyond imagination of expectancy, *samadhi* bliss!
Not an unconscious state
Or mental chloroform without wilful return,
Samadhi but extends my conscious realm
Beyond limits of the mortal frame

Samadhi

To farthest boundary of eternity
Where I, the Cosmic Sea,
Watch the little ego floating in Me.
The sparrow, each grain of sand, fall not without My sight.
All space floats like an iceberg in My mental sea.
Colossal Container, I, of all things made.
By deeper, longer, thirsty, guru-given meditation
Comes this celestial *samadhi*.
Mobile murmurs of atoms are heard,
The dark earth, mountains, vales, lo! molten liquid!
Flowing seas change into vapors of nebulae!
Aum blows upon vapors, opening wondrously their veils,
Oceans stand revealed, shining electrons,
Till, at last sound of the cosmic drum,
Vanish the grosser lights into eternal rays
Of all-pervading bliss.
From joy I came, for joy I live, in sacred joy I melt.
Ocean of mind, I drink all creation's waves.
Four veils of solid, liquid, vapor, light,
Lift aright.
Myself, in everything, enters the Great Myself.
Gone forever, fitful, flickering shadows of mortal memory.
Spotless is my mental sky, below, ahead, and high above.
Eternity and I, one united ray.
A tiny bubble of laughter, I
Am become the Sea of Mirth Itself.*

---

* Paramhansa Yogananda, *Autobiography of a Yogi* (Nevada City, California: Crystal Clarity Publishers, 2005), 146–47.

Epilogue

Two Bears Crossing

"We send thanks to all the animal life in the world. They have many things to teach us as people. We are glad they are still here, and we hope it will always be so."

—Excerpt from a Mohawk Indian
Thanksgiving Address to a new America

Spring 2017

IT IS 2:17 IN the morning and I cannot sleep. When this happens, I rise and sneak into our meditation room to dive into the cool and electrifying states of inner sanctuary. Not tonight. I am writing a note to you.

Nakula is in a different realm, snoring contentedly after a day spent working on the Karuna Sagara land across from Ananda. Earlier in the day I went to find him. I drove up the hill towards a knoll where fifty of us had blessed the land on March 7, 2016, sixty-four years after Yogananda's mahasamadhi. Sacred space for a small temple, hand-built by young adults, dedicated to yoga meditation.

The land will be for a new generation of yogis, our children, other children who want to live simply in a small community, with a view towards higher consciousness. Their way would be different yet similar. At some point we must let go and let them find their own way, their own voice. It is my sincere desire that love for God will reign foremost on this land. Kriya Yoga and devotion to God are the future.

The spring rains have been abundant, suffusing the earth in hope and new growth. The large pond behind the new land is full. I stop the car and walk out, looking for him. In the distance I see an old backhoe tractor, its stabilizers up in the air like some upside-down beetle. Nakula is gazing at a huge tree stump that has been turned on one side, its twirling roots creating a sculpture more stunning than any artist could image. I sense what he is thinking.

After taking seclusion on the land he had asked Divine Mother how we could find the money to build here. He sent up an urgent prayer. Then he looked around and inwardly heard the trees answer: 'Don't worry, use us!' They were offering themselves to help build a small community.

Soon after, the electric company needed to cut a swath of trees through our land to make way for a new line that would travel deep into the forest of the High Sierras. When Nakula told the tree removal crew that he had a use for the logs from the trees, the crew hauled the logs up the hill and stacked them near the sacred spot where the temple was to be.

Nearby was a small temple dedicated to Hanuman* that Nakula had built when we first bought the land. Hanuman loves the forest; in India his temples are often surrounded by trees. The temple is tiny, only three feet high and two feet wide, and with a pointed roof. As a symbol that the land is home to a swami, we positioned a triangular red flag from India. Inside we placed a small Hanuman statue belonging to our son, Rama. Friends brought photos of saints, gurus, gods, and goddesses.

Most of the workers that cleared the trees were Mexican gentlemen with little English. We noticed that after they finished clearing the trees they had left several coins at the Hanuman Shrine. It was their way of adding blessings to the land and the coming community.

As I walked towards Nakula, I called his name. Finally, as I came closer, he whirled around and walked towards me. "Did you see them, did you see the

---

* Hanuman is one of the legendary heroes of the Ramayana, an ancient Hindu epic scripture.

bears?" His voice was excited. My thoughts raced. *A whole clan of bears? Five bears, what bears was he talking about?*

He walked right up to me. "Did you see the bears?" he asked again. I answered him with my thoughts. *No, I did not see the bears. What bears?* Black bear sightings were rare these days and he knew my concerns that their habitat was shrinking.

He had been using his tractor to clear a small path on the land. He gestured up the hill. "They were right there, right on the path." He led me through the forest to an area where brush had been cleared. The dirt was orange and copper, thick mud churned by a long winter and spring of heavy rainfall. After five years of drought, Mother Nature had inundated the earth.

"See, right over there, that's where I saw them. They came right out of the bushes and crossed in front of me, right here." He was looking at the ground and couldn't contain his excitement. "There were two of them. The larger one was huge, I think the biggest bear I've ever seen. The other was a smaller bear, but it was not a cub. Maybe it was a grown teenager or a young adult." I looked at him in silence.

"The big older bear had a bit of white on its shoulder area." He gestured to indicate it was somewhere between his shoulders and his ears. "As it crossed in front of me, the big one looked right at me." *Bear medicine.*

Nakula turned and waved towards the northeast. "They headed down through the bushes, right there towards the pond." He walked over to a muddy ledge. "See? You can see their prints right here."

We both looked down. On the ground below were several prints where their large paws had sunk into the thick mud.

"Two bears crossing," I said. "They are blessing the land. They are still here."

A few years back, when we first walked the land, I had seen bear scat. It was on a trail so steep that I had had to climb on hands and knees. Even at the Meditation Retreat I had not seen a bear for several years, since right before the worst of the drought.

Sometimes at the retreat I would hear gunshots. A neighbor a few miles from us explained: "Oh, that's a guy that likes to shoot for target practice, and to scare the bears from his compost."

All this time the wild black bears have been hiding from us—they are really quite timid.

"Are we encroaching on their habitat?" I asked Nakula. "Why, yes!" he almost shouted.

I sighed. *We must let them know that we won't harm them. We must send them our love. We must be careful how we live. They will be crossing here again, to get to the pond.*

Morning is coming. On the table in front of me is the printout of a Vedic astrological chart. Melanie, a young yoga teacher, twenty-six, female. Pisces rising, moon in Taurus, an exalted Jupiter in Cancer. Saturn in Capricorn. It was the chart of a healer and a teacher. "A lovely chart," my astrologer friend had commented.

It is four in the morning and I walk upstairs to hear a few cries from our family cat, now nineteen and firmly in his last stage of life. He is sleeping in the soft bed we made for him. I reach down and scratch his chin and ears. "You're a good boy, we love you." I give him a bit of food and he settles down again. He can no longer move like he used to and avoids climbing stairs. He depends on us to care for him.

The sun will be up soon. I move onto the deck to recite the Gayatri Mantra, then energize.

A few barks in the distance. Is it a coyote or a neighbor's dog?

A friend recently asked what the world will look like in one hundred years. I laughed and thought: *It's not going to be like anything we can imagine.*

Resources

To receive healing prayers for yourself or others: prayers@ananda.org

To visit the Crystal Hermitage Gardens:
crystalhermitage.org/gardens/

Yogic schools for youth (see chapter four, Student stage):
the Education for Life Foundation offers both online and in-person
Teacher Training: edforlife.org

Family Yoga retreats, youth camps at Ananda Village:
anandavillage.org

Ananda University currently offers online programs:
anandauniversity.org. The Conference for Precession and Ancient
Knowledge (CPAK) meets every other year: cycleoftheages.org

To learn about Kriya Yoga: ananda.org/kriya-yoga/

Spiritual pilgrimages: The Expanding Light offers sacred pilgrimages.
Ananda Italy and Ananda India also offer pilgrimages.

To learn more about yoga, meditation, yoga therapy, yoga teacher
training or meditation teacher training, or to bring a group, visit
expandinglight.org

To visit the Ananda Meditation Retreat for yourself or your group: meditationretreat.org

Nischala Cryer occasionally leads retreats for groups focusing on aspects of the Four Stages of Yoga: meditationretreat@ananda.org; or nischala@anandauniversity.org

Internships for Young Adults: anandavillage.org/internships

Yogananda's meditation techniques, free support: ananda.org/meditation

Ananda yoga communities can be found in Italy, near the town of Assisi; at Ananda Village outside of Nevada City, California; and in the following cities: Palo Alto, California; Seattle, Washington; Portland, Oregon; Sacramento, California; and Pune, India. Meditation groups, online virtual yoga community: ananda.org; Ananda Europa/Italy: ananda.it; Ananda India: anandaindia.org

About the Author

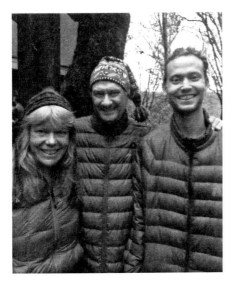

NISCHALA CRYER LIVES WITH her family at a remote meditation retreat in the Sierra Nevada foothills outside of Nevada City, California. She is co-founder of Ananda University, a unique school offering "higher education for higher consciousness." In the mid-eighties she traded corporate life for living in a spiritual community. She is author of *Reflections on Living 30 Years in a Spiritual Community*.

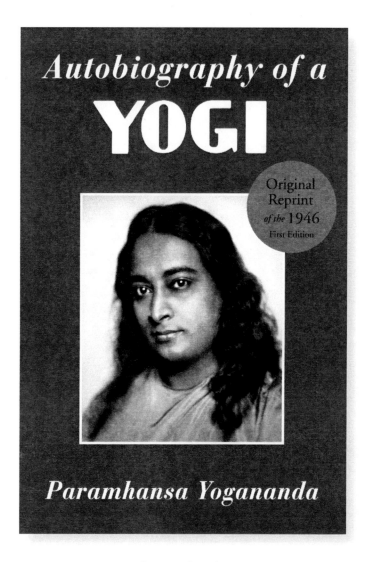

Autobiography of a Yogi
Paramhansa Yogananda

Autobiography of a Yogi is one of the best-selling Eastern philosophy titles of all time, with millions of copies sold, named one of the best and most influential books of the twentieth century. This highly prized reprinting of the original 1946 edition is the only one available free from textual changes made after Yogananda's death. Yogananda was the first yoga master of India whose mission was to live and teach in the West.

Also available in unabridged audiobook (MP3) format, read by Swami Kriyananda.